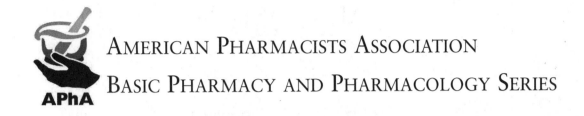

AMERICAN PHARMACISTS ASSOCIATION
BASIC PHARMACY AND PHARMACOLOGY SERIES

Pharmacy Technician

WORKBOOK AND CERTIFICATION REVIEW

-SECOND EDITION-

PERSPECTIVE PRESS
MORTON PUBLISHING COMPANY
www.morton-pub.com

Morton Publishing

Printed in the United States of America.

Morton Publishing Company
925 West Kenyon Avenue, Unit 12
Englewood, CO 80110
phone: 1-303-761-4805
fax: 1-303-762-9923

International Standard Book Number
0-89582-651-8

10 9 8 7 6 5 4 3 2

PHARMACY TECHNICIAN

WORKBOOK AND
CERTIFICATION REVIEW

SECOND EDITION

TABLE OF CONTENTS

TABLE OF CONTENTS

ACKNOWLEDGEMENTS

Mary F. Powers, Ph.D., R.Ph.

Mary Powers was a key contributor to both the first and second editions of **The Pharmacy Technician**, on which this workbook is based; was a key contributor to the first edition of this workbook; and has played an expanded role in the development of the second edition of both texts. For the second edition of the **Pharmacy Technician Workbook and Certification Review** Mary collaborated with the publisher on a plan for the new edition, updated existing content to reflect changes made in the corresponding text, updated and expanded the Practice Exam, and provided a wealth of new material including a new Calculations Practice Exam, new multiple choice questions for each chapter, additional prescription and medication order exercises, and new In the Workplace tools and activities to help students check their knowledge and practice their skills. An Associate Professor of Pharmacy Practice at the University of Toledo College of Pharmacy, Toledo, OH., Mary's input was enormously helpful.

Joe Medina, CPhT, B.S. Pharmacy

Joe Medina contributed to the first edition of this Workbook and Review by writing many of the exam review questions and other exercises. Joe has served as the Chairperson/Program Director for the Pharmacy Technician Programs at Front Range Community College and Arapahoe Community College in the Denver metro area.

Others We'd Like To Thank

This workbook would also not have been possible without the efforts of a large number of people who worked on the corresponding text, **The Pharmacy Technician, Second Edition**. I'd like to thank them again for their contributions to that book and mention them as well. We couldn't have done it without their help:

Robert P. Shrewsbury, Ph.D., R.Ph., Associate Professor of Pharmaceutics, University of North Carolina-Chapel Hill; Brenda Hanneson Vondereau, B.Sc. (Pharm.), Clinical Services Pharmacist, Catalyst Rx; Cindy Johnson, R.Ph., MSW, Pharmacist, Colorado Mental Health Institute; Betsy A. Gilman, Pharm.D, Director, Singac Pharmacy.; and Pamela Nicoski, Pharm.D., Clinical Pharmacist, Loyola University Medical Center.

In addition to the contributors we are grateful to several reviewers whose insights and feedback on the first edition helped shape the second edition: James Austin, Weatherford College; Marisa Fetzer, Institute of Technology; Claudia Johnson, Polytech Adult Education; Mary Anna Marshall, Richmond Apothecaries, Virginia Institute for Pharmacy Technicians, J. Sargent Reynolds Community College, and the Virginia Pharmacists Association; Peter Vondereau, Scolan's Pharmacy; and Walgreen Co.

We would also like to thank two great artists, Tammy Newnam and Anna Veltfort; and Doug Morton, whose sponsorship makes this book possible. Finally, I'd like to thank my family for their help, support and patience.

—Alison Reeves

PREFACE

THIS WORKBOOK

This workbook was developed to correspond with the textbook, **The Pharmacy Technician** by Perspective Press. For pharmacy technician students, it is a valuable tool for success in your training course. It provides a useful format for memorizing important information and for checking your knowledge of it. Key concepts and terms are carefully explained, and there are over 1000 exercises and problems to test your knowledge. Working these exercises out successfully will help you to succeed in your training.

It is important you follow through the workbook chapter by chapter and try answering the questions before looking up the answers. Once you have completed a chapter, review it and try to memorize the answers to the questions you missed.

A REVIEW GUIDE

The workbook can also be used as a review guide in preparing for the National Pharmacy Technician Certification Examination. All its chapters are important in the taking of the National Exam. However, special attention should be placed on Chapter 6 - Calculations, as the exam will have calculation type problem solving that is often challenging for technicians taking the exam. The method used (ratio & proportion) in this section will solve any calculation problem you come across on the National Certification Examination as well as most problems in the pharmacy setting. A careful review of this workbook will prepare you for much of the national exam. However, some questions on that exam require knowledge gained from practice as a technician. Pharmacy technicians who have work experience in a pharmacy setting will therefore have an advantage in taking the National Exam. As an additional study tool, we have included a practice exam at the back of this book in the same *choose the best answer* format of the national exam.

OVERVIEW: PHARMACY TECHNICIAN CERTIFICATION EXAM

The National Pharmacy Technician Certification Examination was established to allow the certification of technicians. The need for highly qualified pharmacy technicians is increasingly important as pharmacists are relinquishing many dispensing duties for more clinical ones, and the technician is playing a greater role.

Currently the national examination is given by the Pharmacy Technician Certification Board (PTCB) and is offered three times a year in the months of March, July, and November. Applications for the taking of this examination must be made two months prior to the scheduled exam day. The cost of taking this examination is at the time of this writing one-hundred and twenty dollars.

THE EXAM

The examination contains 125 multiple choice questions plus an additional 15 non-scored items, for a total of 140 questions. These questions are derived from a data base of several thousand questions. Therefore, examinations given on certain dates are not the same as ones given on a different date. The multiple choice format involves four possible answers with only one answer being the best or most correct. The time limit for taking this examination is three hours.

PREFACE

SCORING OF EXAM

The scoring of the examination is based on the combined average of scores in three functional areas:

1. Assisting the Pharmacist in Serving Patients (64% of Exam)

   Includes activities related to traditional pharmacy prescription dispensing and medication distribution, and collecting and organizing information.

2. Maintaining Medication and Inventory Control Systems (25% of Exam)

   Includes activities related to medication and supply purchasing, inventory control, and preparation and distribution of medications according to approved policies and procedures.

3. Participating in the Administration and Management of Pharmacy Practice (11% of Exam)

   Includes activities related to the administrative process for the pharmacy practice center, including: operations, human resources, facilities and equipment, and information systems.

The combined score range of the exam is 300 to 900 points with a passing of 650 points required.

WHAT YOU NEED TO KNOW FOR THE EXAM

Specific information on examination content is provided in the PTCB's **Guidebook to Certification**, which can be downloaded from their site: www.ptcb.org. In general, the examination tests:

➥ *knowledge of the role of the pharmacy technician in the pharmacy (i.e., prescriptions, legal issues, compounding, etc.)*. This workbook provides an excellent overview of this area, and for technicians with work experience, your experience on the job should reinforce it.

➥ *knowledge of the most commonly used drugs (including trade and generic names, indications, etc.)*. Since the pharmacy technician is not responsible for the counseling patients, this section is limited in the number of questions presented on the exam. Job experience and Appendix A of this workbook are a good preparation.

➥ *ability to perform common calculations (for a specific dose, for additives in IV solutions, for ml/minute and gtt/minute, etc.)*. As a result, it's a good idea to thoroughly study the calculation section of this workbook.

For additional information, contact the PTCB at:

Pharmacy Technician Certification Board
2215 Constitution Avenue, NW
Washington, DC 20037-2985
202-429-7576
http://www.ptcb.org

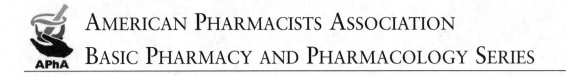

Dear Student or Instructor,

The American Pharmacists Association (APhA), the national professional society of pharmacists in the United States, and Morton Publishing Company, a publisher of educational texts and training materials in healthcare, are pleased to present this outstanding workbook, *Pharmacy Technician Workbook and Certification Review, Second Edition.* It is one of a series of distinctive texts and training materials for basic pharmacy and pharmacology training that is published under this banner: *American Pharmacists Association Basic Pharmacy and Pharmacology Series.*

Each book in the series is oriented toward developing an understanding of fundamental concepts. In addition, each text presents applied and practical information on the skills necessary to function effectively in the workplace. Each of the books in the series uses a visual design to enhance understanding and ease of use and is accompanied by various instructional support materials. We think you will find them valuable training tools.

The American Pharmacists Association and Morton Publishing thank you for using this book and invite you to look at other titles in this series, which are listed below.

John A. Gans, PharmD
Executive Vice President
American Pharmacists Association

Douglas N. Morton
President
Morton Publishing Company

OTHER TITLES IN THIS SERIES:

The Pharmacy Technician, Second Edition
Basic Pharmacology
Drug Card Workbook

NOTICE

To the best of the Publisher's knowledge, the information presented in this book follows general practice as well as federal and state regulations and guidelines. However, please note that you are responsible for following your employer's and your state's policies and guidelines.

The job description for pharmacy technicians varies by institution and state. Your employer and state can provide you with the most recent regulations, guidelines, and practices that apply to your work.

The Publisher of this book disclaims any responsibility whatsoever for any injuries, damages, or other conditions that result from your practice of the skills described in this book for any reason whatsoever.

– 1 –

PHARMACY AND HEALTH CARE

KEY CONCEPTS

Test your knowledge by covering the information in the right hand column.

pharmacology	The study of drugs, their properties, uses, application and effects.
herbal medicine	People have used drugs derived from plants to treat illnesses and other physical conditions for thousands of years. The ancient Greeks used the bark of a white willow tree to relieve pain. The bark contained salicylic acid, the natural forerunner of the active ingredient in aspirin.
cocaine	The first effective local anesthetic.
digitalis	The drug of the foxglove plant which has been widely used in treating heart disease.
quinine	The first useful drug in the treatment of malaria, one of mankind's most deadly diseases. It was extracted from the bark of a Peruvian tree, the Cinchona.
germ theory	The theory that microorganisms cause food spoilage.
polio vaccine	The use of an injectable vaccine made from killed polio virus and an oral polio vaccine made from a weakened form of live polio virus was important to prevent the spread of this crippling and often fatal disease.
insulin	The hormone that lowers blood sugar in the treatment of diabetes–one of the great discoveries in medicine in the twentieth century.

penicillin	The first antibiotic.
average life span	This measure of health has increased by over twenty years in the United States in the Twentieth Century.
synthetic drugs	Drugs created by reformulating simpler chemicals into more complex ones, creating a new chemical not found in nature.
Human Genome Project	An attempt to map the entire DNA sequence in the human genome. This information will provide a better understanding of hereditary diseases and how to treat them.
pharmacist education and training	In the United States, an individual must graduate from an accredited college of pharmacy, pass a state licensing exam, and perform an internship working under a licensed pharmacist. Once licensed, the pharmacist must receive continuing education to maintain their license.
cost control	A significant trend in recent health care has been the effort to control the cost of prescription drugs, on aspect of which is the use of closed "formularies" that rely substantially on substituting generic drugs in place of more expensive brands.
computerization	Pharmacy computer systems put customer profiles, product, inventory, pricing, and other essential information within easy access. One result has been that pharmacies and pharmacists dispense more prescriptions and information than ever before.

STUDY NOTES

Use this area to write important points you'd like to remember.

FILL IN THE KEY TERM

Use these key terms to fill in the correct blank. Answers are at the end of the book.

antibiotic	hormone	panacea
antitoxin	human genome	Paracelsus
Shen Nung	managed care	pharmaceutical
data	materia medica	pharmacology
formularies	OBRA '90	salicylic acid

1. _____ : an ancient practitioner of "trial and error" drug testing through tasting plants and other natural materials to determine which were poisonous and which were beneficial.

2. _____ : the natural drug derived from the bark of a white willow tree, used by the Ancient Greeks to relieve pain, and the natural forerunner to the active ingredient in aspirin.

3. _____ : an authoritative listing of drugs and issues related to their use.

4. _____ : of or about drugs; also, a drug product.

5. _____ : a cure-all.

6. _____ : the study of drugs—their properties, uses, application, and effects.

7. _____ : he is generally credited with firmly establishing the use of chemistry to create medicinal drugs.

8. _____ : the information stored in a computer.

9. _____ : a substance that acts against a toxin in the body.

10. _____ : a substance which harms or kills microorganisms like bacteria and fungi.

11. _____ : chemicals produced by the body that regulate body functions and processes.

12. _____ : the complete set of genetic material contained in a human cell.

13. _____ : U.S. legislation which required pharmacists to provide consulting services to Medicaid patients.

14. _____ : lists of drugs that are approved for use by patients.

15. _____ : a major factor contributing to the attempt to control costs of prescription drugs.

TRUE/FALSE

Indicate whether the statement is true or false in the blank. Answers are at the end of the book.

_____ 1. The natural drug that is the forerunner to aspirin comes from the cinchona tree.

_____ 2. Almost all drugs used today are made synthetically.

_____ 3. Digitalis comes from the foxglove plant.

_____ 4. Cocaine was the first general anesthetic.

_____ 5. The average life span in the U.S. increased over 50% in the twentieth century.

_____ 6. More pharmacists and technicians are employed in community pharmacies than in any other setting.

_____ 7. The second largest area of employment for pharmacists and technicians is home care.

_____ 8. The pharmacist is generally considered the second most trusted professional, behind doctors.

_____ 9. The use of generic drugs is a major trend in the effort to cut the costs of medication.

_____ 10. Pharmacy computer systems prevent mistakes in data entry.

EXPLAIN WHY

Explain why these statements are true or important. Check your answers in the text. Discuss any questions you may have with your Instructor.

1. Give at least three reasons why synthetic drugs are important.

2. Why was the use of anesthesia revolutionary?

3. Why was Paracelsus's work important?

4. Why was penicillin a major benefit in wartime?

5. Why is the Human Genome Project important to pharmacology?

6. Why are drug patents important?

7. Why are pharmacists among the most trusted professionals?

CHOOSE THE BEST ANSWER

Answers are at the end of the book.

1. The drug digitalis comes from the foxglove plant and is used to treat some _____ conditions.
   a. liver
   b. kidney
   c. heart
   d. lung

2. The first publicized operation using general anesthesia was performed using _____ as the anesthetic
   a. cocaine
   b. foxglove
   c. quinine
   d. ether

3. The field of _____ has resulted from the study of the human genome.
   a. pharmacology
   b. biotechnology
   c. natural medicine
   d. discovery

4. Quinine comes from the bark of the cinchona and was used to treat
   a. malaria.
   b. diabetes.
   c. heart disease.
   d. hypertension.

5. The ancient Greek god of Medicine was
   a. Imhotep
   b. Zeus
   c. Aseculapius
   d. Panacea

6. _____ advocated "bleeding" to maintain balance of the "humours."
   a. Charaka
   b. Shen Nung
   c. Pontos
   d. Galen

7. _____ showed that an extract of insulin could lower blood sugar in dogs.
   a. Watson and Crick
   b. Banting and Best
   c. Fleming
   d. Hippocrates

STUDY NOTES

Use this area to write important points you'd like to remember.

— 2 —

THE PHARMACY TECHNICIAN

KEY CONCEPTS

Test your knowledge by covering the information in the right hand column.

job responsibilities

Pharmacy technicians perform essential tasks that do not require the pharmacist's skill or expertise. Specific responsibilities and tasks differ by setting and are described in writing by each employer through job descriptions, policy and procedure manuals, and other documents.

supervision

Pharmacy technicians work under the direct supervision of a licensed pharmacist who is legally responsible for their performance.

pharmacist counseling

Having technicians assist the pharmacist frees the pharmacist for activities which require a greater level of expertise, such as counseling with patients.

scope of practice

What individuals may and may not do in their jobs is often referred to as their "scope of practice."

employment opportunities

Like pharmacists, most pharmacy technicians are employed in community pharmacies and hospitals. However, they are also employed in clinics, home care, long term care, mail order prescription pharmacies, and various other settings.

specialized jobs

In various hospital and other environments, there are specialized technician jobs which require more advanced skills developed from additional education, training and experience.

trustworthiness

Pharmacy technicians are entrusted with confidential patient information, dangerous substances, and perishable products.

errors

Drugs, whether prescription or over the counter, can be dangerous if misused, and mistakes by pharmacy technicians can be life-threatening.

Health Insurance Portability and Accountability Act (HIPAA)	Pharmacy technicians are legally responsible for the privacy and security of protected health information (PHI).
math skills	Pharmacy technicians routinely perform mathematical calculations in filling prescriptions and other activities.
terminology	Pharmacy technicians must learn the specific pharmaceutical terminology that will be used on the job.
teamwork	Pharmacy technicians must be able to communicate, cooperate, and work effectively with others.
standards	There is no federal standard for pharmacy technician training or competency. However there are state and employer standards which must be met.
certification	A valuable career step for pharmacy technicians is getting certification by an appropriate organization or body. It verifies an individual's competence as a technician, and indicates a high level of knowledge and skill. In the United States, the Pharmacy Technician Certification Board (PTCB) provides technician national certification.

STUDY NOTES

Use this area to write important points you'd like to remember.

IN THE WORKPLACE

These sample job descriptions may help you in your career choice.

Sample Pharmacy Technician Job Description—Community Pharmacy

General Definition

The purpose of the pharmacy technician is to assist the pharmacist with the day-do-day activities in the pharmacy.

Responsibilities

- Help patients who are dropping off or picking up prescription orders
- Enter prescription orders into the computer
- Create a profile of the patient's health and insurance information in the computer or update the patient's profile
- Communicate with insurance carriers to obtain payment for prescription claims
- Complete weekly distribution center medication orders, place orders on shelves, and verify all associated paperwork
- Assist the pharmacist with filling and labeling prescriptions
- Prepare the pharmacy for inventory
- Screen telephone calls for the pharmacist
- Communicate with prescribers and their agents to obtain refill authorization
- Compound oral solutions, ointments, and creams
- Prepackage bulk medications

Qualifications

- Professional demeanor
- Ability to respect confidentiality of patient data
- Strong communication skills
- Courteous attitude
- Understanding of medical terminology and calculations
- Ability to type at least 35 words per minute
- Knowledge of computer operations
- Knowledge of medication brand and generic names
- Knowledge of insurance and third-party payment systems
- High school diploma or graduate equivalent degree
- National certification desirable

Sample Pharmacy Technician Job Description—Hospital Pharmacy

General Definition

Under the direction of a pharmacist, the pharmacy technician performs pharmacy-related functions, in compliance with department policies and procedures, that provide optimal pharmaceutical care.

Responsibilities

- Rotate through all work areas of the pharmacy
- Transport medications, drug-delivery devices, and other pharmacy equipment from the pharmacy to nursing units and clinics
- Pick up copies of physician orders, automated medication administration records, and unused medications from the nursing units and return them to the pharmacy
- Fill patient medication cassettes
- Prepare medications and supplies for dispensing, including:
  —prepackaging bulk medications
  —compounding ointments, creams, oral solutions, and other medications
  —preparing chemotherapeutic agents
  —compounding total parenteral nutrition solutions
  —compounding large-volume intravenous mixtures
  —packaging and preparing drugs being used in clinical investigations
  —preparing prescriptions for outpatients
- Assist pharmacists in entering medication orders into the computer system
- Prepare inventories, order drugs and supplies from the storeroom, receive drugs, and stock shelves in various pharmacy locations
- Screen telephone calls
- Perform monthly nursing unit inspections, maintain workload records, and collect quality-assurance data
- Assist in training new employees
- Assist other pharmacy technicians

Qualifications

- Valid state pharmacy technician registration (required in some states)
- High school diploma or graduate equivalent degree
- National certification desirable

Training and Experience

Must have one year of hospital pharmacy experience, have completed a pharmacy technician vocational course, or be a pharmacy student

Knowledge and Skills

- Ability to work as a team member
- Good communication skills
- Knowledge of basic pharmacy practices and procedures
- Knowledge of medications and medical supplies
- Strong mathematical computation skills
- Knowledge of record-keeping techniques
- Attention to detail
- Accurate typing skills (minimum 35 words per minute)
- Basic understanding of computer technology

Source: Reproduced by permission from *The Pharmacy Technician Companion: Your Road Map to Technician Training and Careers* (Washington, D.C. American Pharmaceutical Association, 1998), pp. 9-10. © 1998 by the American Pharmaceutical Association.

Certified Pharmacy Technician Managed Care - Job Description

Job Title: Certified Pharmacy Technician – Managed Care

Education:
Nationally Certified Pharmacy Technician (CPhT) – Required;
High School Graduate – Required;
Business/College Courses – Preferred;
Medical Terminology Courses – Preferred.

Qualifications:
Strong organizational, prioritization, communications & mathematics skills – Required;
Pharmacy Claims Processing Computer System experience – Preferred;
Minimum 2 years experience in a retail pharmacy setting and/or managed care/pharmacy benefit environment;
Comprehensive understanding of third party pharmacy benefit plan parameters;
Ability to understand the importance of and respect the confidentiality of all patient information;

Computer Literacy with proficiency in general word-processing and data entry.

Duties:
Under the supervision of a pharmacist: daily handling of on-going pharmacy benefit telephone calls from members, pharmacy providers & physicians;
Troubleshooting third party prescription claims questions with an understanding of on-line rejections and plan parameters;
Developing and maintaining an electronic service log on all telephone calls with complete follow-up history;
Developing a trending report on the aforementioned service calls with an eye towards forecasting possible trends in pharmacy service;
Providing as needed telephone and administrative support for the department.

Hours: TBA

Reports to: Managed Care Supervisor

Source: Reproduced by permission from the Pharmacy Technician Certification Board website at http://www.ptcb.org. © Copyright Pharmacy Technician Certification Board.

IN THE WORKPLACE

These sample resumes may help you when applying for a position as a pharmacy technician.

Résumé 1   **Actual résumé size is 8.5 x 11**

This résumé is for a pharmacy technician looking at career options in community pharmacy. It shows the inclusion of high school education when college studies have not been completed.

Ashley Brooke Foster

Local Address	Permanent Address
9501 Rio Verde Way	3301 Thorntree Road
Tucson, Arizona 85710	Scottsville, Arizona 85260
(480) 451-8142	(520) 290-7721
E-mail:abfoster@u.arizona.edu	

OBJECTIVE: To obtain a pharmacy technician position in a community pharmacy

EDUCATION:

University of Arizona	August 1999 – Present
Tucson, Arizona	Graduation Anticipated: 2003
Major: B.S. in Chemistry	G.P.A.: 3.4 / 4.0
Chaparral High School	September 1995 – May 1999
Scottsville, Arizona	

EXPERIENCE:

Hazleton Realtors	June 1999 – August 1999
Scottsville, Arizona	
Receptionist	
Johnson Floral Designs	May 1998 – August 1998
Scottsville, Arizona	
Sales Associate	
Verda Country Club	June 1997 – August 1997
Scottsville, Arizona	
Lifeguard	
Mary Immaculate Hospital	July 1996 – December 1998
Scottsville, Arizona	
Volunteer (4-20 Hours/Week)	

CERTIFICATES:

American Red Cross First Aid Certificate	1997 - 2000
American Red Cross Adult CPR Certificate	1997 - 2000
American Red Cross Infant & Child CPR	1997 - 2000

MEMBERSHIPS:

Student Affiliates of the American	1999 - Present
Chemical Society and Chemistry Club	
University of Arizona	

Résumé 2   Actual résumé size is 8.5 x 11

This is another résumé format for a pharmacy technician. This person is attending college, but is not necessarily carrying a full academic load.

Page A. Shaw
3321 Guyton Way, Apartment 32A
Jacksonville, Florida 32225
904/645-9729

EDUCATION

September 1996 – Present (Part-time)	University of North Florida College of Arts and Sciences Jacksonville, Florida Completed 44 Semester Hours
September 1992 – May 1996	Providence High School Jacksonville, Florida

WORK EXPERIENCE

July 1996 – Present	Eckerd Pharmacy, Jacksonville, FL Pharmacy Technician Assist pharmacists in performing tasks and duties related to dispensing prescription medications
May 1995 – August 1995	Sunshine Gallery, Inc., Atlantic Beach, FL Customer Service Clerk Sold, matted and framed art work
May 1994 – August 1994	Jackson and Associates, Atlantic Beach, FL Secretarial Assistant Performed general administrative tasks
May 1993 – September 1993	Leed's Department Store, Jacksonville, FL Sales Associate Responsible for the sale of children's clothing

COMPUTER SKILLS

Microsoft Windows, Word, Excel, Access; WordPerfect

ORGANIZATIONS

January 1997 – Present	Pre-Medical Professsion's Program University of North Florida

REFERENCES

Provided upon request

Source: Reproduced by permission from *The Pharmacy Professional's Guide to Résumés, CV's & Interviewing* (Washington, D.C. American Pharmaceutical Association, 2001), pp. 18-21. © Copyright 2001 by the American Pharmaceutical Association.

These sample resumes may help you when applying for a position as a pharmacy technician.

Résumé 3

Actual résumé size is 8.5 x 11

A résumé of a pharmacy technician majoring in pre-pharmacy and seeking a change in practice experience.

MICHAEL PATRICK GARRETT

804-A Westside Avenue • Iowa City, Iowa 52240 • 319.358.5107
E-mail: mpgarret@uiowa.edu

OBJECTIVE	Pharmacy technician position in a health-system pharmacy	
EDUCATION	August 1999 - Present	University of Iowa Iowa City, Iowa Major: Pre-Pharmacy
	September 1998 – May 1999	Grand View College Des Moines, Iowa
WORK EXPERIENCE	JUNE 1999 – AUGUST 1999	PHARMACY TECHNICIAN Albertson's Pharmacy Des Moines, Iowa Supervisor: Ted Hankle, R.Ph. 319.785.6700
	MAY 1994 – AUGUST 1998 (Summers)	GROUNDSKEEPER Deer Valley Golf Club Des Moines, Iowa Supervisor: James Simpson 319.472.8739
HONORS	Dean's List, Grand View College, Spring 1999 Eagle Scout, Mid-Iowa Council, 1996	
REFERENCES	Upon request	

Source: Reproduced by permission from *The Pharmacy Professional's Guide to Résumés, CV's & Interviewing* (Washington, D.C. American Pharmaceutical Association, 2001), pp. 18-21. © Copyright 2001 by the American Pharmaceutical Association.

Résumé 4   Actual résumé size is 8.5 x 11

A résumé of a career pharmacy technician.

MINH T. NGO

5231 Warfield Drive
Oakland, CA 94611
(510) 339-5416

_____EXPERIENCE_____

June 1999 – Present	Pharmacy Technician	Bayside Pharmacy Oakland, CA
May 1998 – August 1998	Pharmacy Technician	Providence Hospital Oakland, CA
June 1997 – August 1997	Bank Teller	Wells Fargo Bank Berkeley, CA
July 1995 – December 1998 (10 -30 Hours / Week)	Waiter / Cook	Great Wall Restaurant Berkeley, CA

_____EDUCATION_____

September 1995 – June 1999	Freemont High School Oakland, California	Diploma

_____CERTIFICATES_____

1998 – Present	Certified Pharmacy Technician	Successfully Completed Pharmacy Technician Certification Board Exam

_____COMMUNITY SERVICE_____

January 1997 – Present (8 Hours / Month)	Volunteer	Metropolitan Area Food Bank Oakland, CA

_____REFERENCES_____

Furnished Upon Request

Source: Reproduced by permission from _The Pharmacy Professional's Guide to Résumés, CV's & Interviewing_ (Washington, D.C. American Pharmaceutical Association, 2001), pp. 18-21. © Copyright 2001 by the American Pharmaceutical Association.

FILL IN THE KEY TERM

Use these key terms to fill in the correct blank. Answers are at the end of the book.

certification	detail oriented	pharmacist
competent	on-the-job training	professionals
confidentiality	patient rights	scope of practice
counseling	patient welfare	technicians
continuing education	personal inventory	

1. _____ : what individuals may and may not do in their jobs.

2. _____ : to assess characteristics, skills, qualities, etc.

3. _____ : the requirement of health care providers to keep all patient information private among the patient, the patient's insurer, and the providers directly involved in the patient's care.

4. _____ : the most important consideration in health care.

5. _____ : being qualified and capable to perform a task or job.

6. _____ : a legal proof or document that an individual meets certain objective standards, usually provided by a neutral professional organization.

7. _____ : individuals who are given a basic level of training designed to help them perform specific tasks.

8. _____ : individuals who receive extensive and advanced levels of education before being allowed to practice, such as physicians and pharmacists.

9. _____ : technicians always work under their direct supervision.

10. _____ : one of the services pharmacists provide.

11. _____ : patients are generally guaranteed the right to privacy, confidentiality, the information necessary for informed consent, and the freedom to refuse treatment.

12. _____ : a highly important personal characteristic for technicians, since mistakes with drugs can be life-threatening.

13. _____ : a critical element in maintaining competency for pharmacy technicians.

14. _____ : an important part of training that exposes technicians to workplace settings.

TRUE/FALSE

Indicate whether the statement is true or false in the blank. Answers are at the end of the book.

_____ 1. Specific technician responsibilities differ by setting and job description.

_____ 2. Technicians may sometimes provide counseling services to patients.

_____ 3. Technicians are not allowed to do any work that might have serious consequences for patients.

_____ 4. Mathematics skills are very important to the pharmacy technician.

_____ 5. It is essential for technicians to have good interpersonal skills.

_____ 6. The U.S. government sets standards for technician training.

_____ 7. Patient information is considered public information.

_____ 8. Employers monitor the performance and competency of technicians on an ongoing basis.

_____ 9. The ASHP has developed a national model curriculum.

_____ 10. Once earned, the CPhT designation applies for life.

EXPLAIN WHY

Explain why these statements are true or important. Check your answers in the text. Discuss any questions you may have with your Instructor.

1. Give at least two reasons technicians must work under the supervision of a pharmacist.

2. Why is knowing your "scope of practice important?"

3. Why is dependability important?

4. Why is it important that pharmacy technicians understand their responsibilities under the 1996 Health Insurance Portability and Accountability Act (HIPAA)?

5. Why should technicians have math skills?

6. Why are interpersonal skills important?

7. Why is certification a good idea for technicians?

8. Why is continuing education valuable for technicians?

CHOOSE THE BEST ANSWER

Answers are at the end of the book.

1. When technicians perform appropriate essential tasks, this allows the pharmacist time for tasks requiring more advanced professional expertise such as
   a. telephoning insurance companies.
   b. consulting with patients.
   c. counting tablets.
   d. ringing the cash register.

2. Taking routine patient information is a duty of the
   a. consultant.
   b. cashier.
   c. pharmacist.
   d. pharmacy technician.

3. Pharmacy technicians should be dependable. This means
   a. technicians' work can always be done by pharmacists.
   b. technicians are not as important as pharmacists.
   c. the patient, the pharmacist, and the patient's health care team will depend on technician to perform his/her job as required, whether or not anyone is observing.
   d. tardiness is acceptable.

4. Do pharmacy technicians need to maintain good physical and mental health?
   a. Yes, to decrease the chance of making serious mistakes.
   b. Yes, because some belong to labor unions.
   c. No. Pharmacists are always responsible for the technician, so technicians don't have to worry about getting enough sleep.
   d) No. Pharmacists have more education and so will catch all errors made.

5. Pharmacy technicians _____ learn the specific language and terminology used on the job
   a. never need to
   b. must
   c. find it is optional to

6. The _____ curriculum provides a national standard for developing pharmacy technician competency.
   a. PTCB
   b. APhA
   c. PTEC
   d. ASHP

7. _____ are regularly scheduled events to monitor and document technician competency.
   a. PTCE
   b. PTCB
   c. Performance reviews
   d. JCAHO

8. _____ is a legal proof or document that an individual meets certain objective standards, usually provided by a neutral professional organization.
   a. Registration
   b. Certification
   c. Documentation
   d. Prior authorization

9. CPhT stands for
   a. Certified Pharmacy Trainer.
   b. Complete Pharmacy Technician.
   c. Certified Pharmacy Technician.
   d. Certified Pharmacist Technician.

10. Up to _____ contact hours of continuing education for CPhTs can occur at the CPhT's practice site every _____ years.
    a. two, two
    b. ten, one
    c. two, one
    d. ten, two

STUDY NOTES

Use this area to write important points you'd like to remember.

–3–

DRUG REGULATION AND CONTROL

KEY CONCEPTS

Test your knowledge by covering the information in the right hand column.

Food and Drug Administration

The leading enforcement agency at the federal level for regulations concerning drug products.

Drug Enforcement Administration

The agency which controls the distribution of drugs that may be easily abused.

Food and Drug Act of 1906

Prohibited interstate commerce in adulterated or misbranded food, drinks, and drugs. Government pre-approval of drugs is required.

1938 Food, Drug and Cosmetic (FDC) Act

In response to the fatal poisoning of 107 people, primarily children, by an untested sulfanilamide concoction, this comprehensive law requires new drugs be shown to be safe before marketing.

1951 Durham-Humphrey Amendment

This law defines what drugs require a prescription by a licensed practitioner and requires them to include this legend on the label: "Caution: Federal Law prohibits dispensing without a prescription."

1962 Kefauver-Harris Amendments

Requires drug manufacturers to provide proof of both safety and effectiveness before marketing the drug.

1970 Poison Prevention Packaging Act

Requires child-proof packaging on all controlled and most prescription drugs dispensed by pharmacies.

1970 Controlled Substances Act (CSA)

The CSA classifies drugs that may be easily abused and restricts their distribution. It is enforced by the Drug Enforcement Administration (DEA) within the Justice Department.

1990 Omnibus Budget Reconciliation Act (OBRA)

Among other things, this act required pharmacists to offer counseling to Medicaid patients regarding medications, effectively putting the common practice into law.

1996 Health Insurance Portability and Accountability Act (HIPAA)	Provided broad and stringent regulations to protect patients' privacy.
placebos	Inactive substances, not real medications, that are used to test the effectiveness of drugs.
new drugs	All new drugs, whether made domestically or imported, require FDA approval before they can be marketed in the United States.
clinical tests	Tests on proposed new drugs (investigational drugs) are "controlled" by comparing the effect of a proposed drug on one group of patients with the effect of a different treatment on other patients.
blind tests	Patients in a trial are always "blind" to the treatment, i.e, they are not told which control group they are in. In a "double-blind" test, neither the patients nor the physicians know what the medication is.
patent protection	A patent for a new drug gives its manufacturer an exclusive right to market the drug for a specific period of time under a brand name. A drug patent is in effect for 17 years from the date of the drug's discovery. The Hatch-Waxman Act of 1984 provided for up to five year extensions of patent protection to the patent holders to make up for time lost while products went through the FDA approval process.
generics	Once a patent for a brand drug expires, other manufacturers may copy the drug and release it under its pharmaceutical or "generic" name.
labels and labeling	All drugs are required to have clear and accurate information for all labels, inserts, packaging, and so on, but there are different information requirements for various categories of drugs.
prescription drug labels	The minimum requirements on prescription labels for most drugs are as follows: name and address of dispenser, prescription serial number, date of prescription or filling, name of prescriber, name of patient, directions for use, and cautionary statements.
NDC (National Drug Code) number	The number assigned by the manufacturer. Each NDC number has three parts or sets of numbers: The first set indicates the manufacturer; the next set indicates the medication, its strength, and dosage form; the last set indicates the package size.

KEY CONCEPTS

Test your knowledge by covering the information in the right hand column.

controlled substances	A drug which has the potential to be abused and for which distribution is controlled by one of five "schedules."
control classifications	Manufacturers must clearly label controlled drugs with their control classification.
DEA number/formula	The number all prescribers of controlled substances are assigned and which must be used on all controlled drug prescriptions. It has two letters followed by seven single-digit numbers, e.g., AB1234563. The **formula** for checking a DEA number on a prescription form is: if the sum of the first, third and fifth digits is added to twice the sum of the second, fourth, and sixth digits, the total should be a number whose last digit is the same as the last digit of the DEA number.
risks of approved drugs	There is always the risk that an approved drug may produce adverse side effects when used on a larger population.
recalls	Recalls are, with a few exceptions, voluntary on the part of the manufacturer. There are three classes of recalls: 1.) where there is a strong likelihood that the product will cause serious adverse effects or death; 2.) where a product may cause temporary but reversible adverse effects, or in which there is little likelihood of serious adverse effects; 3.) where a product is not likely to cause adverse effects.
state regulation	State boards of pharmacy are responsible for licensing all prescribers and dispensers and administering regulations for the practice of pharmacy in the state.
liability	Legal liability means you can be prosecuted for misconduct.
negligence	Failing to do something that should or must be done.

CONTROLLED SUBSTANCE SCHEDULES

The five control schedules are as follows*:

Schedule I:
➡ Each drug has a high potential for abuse and no accepted medical use in the United States. It may not be prescribed. Heroin, various opium derivatives, and hallucinogenic substances are included on this schedule.

Schedule II:
➡ Each drug has a high potential for abuse and may lead to physical or psychological dependence, but also has a currently accepted medical use in the United States. Amphetamines, opium, cocaine, methadone, and various opiates are included on this schedule.

Schedule III:
➡ Each drug's potential for abuse is less than those in Schedules I and II and there is a currently accepted medical use in the U.S., but abuse may lead to moderate or low physical dependence or high psychological dependence. Anabolic steroids and various compounds containing limited quantities of narcotic substances such as codeine are included on this schedule.

Schedule IV:
➡ Each drug has a low potential for abuse relative to Schedule III drugs and there is a current accepted medical use in the U.S., but abuse may lead to limited physical dependence or psychological dependence. Phenobarbital, the sedative chloral hydrate, and the anesthetic methohexital are included in this group.

Schedule V:
➡ Each drug has a low potential for abuse relative to Schedule IV drugs and there is a current accepted medical use in the U.S., but abuse may lead to limited physical dependence or psychological dependence. Compounds containing limited amounts of a narcotic such as codeine are included in this group.

*21 USC Sec. 812. Note: these schedules are revised periodically. It is important to refer to the most current schedule.

Controlled-Substance Prescriptions

Controlled-substance prescriptions have greater requirements at both federal and state levels than other prescriptions, particularly Schedule II drugs. On controlled substance prescriptions, the DEA number must appear on the form and the patient's full street address must be entered.

On Schedule II prescriptions, the form must be signed by the prescriber. In many states, there are specific time limits that require Schedule II prescriptions be promptly filled. Generally, quantities are limited and no refills are allowed.

Federal requirements for Schedules III-V are less stringent than for Schedule II. *For example, Schedules III-V prescriptions may be refilled up to five times within six months.* However, state and other regulations may be stricter than federal requirements, so it is necessary to know the requirements for your specific job setting.

FILL IN THE KEY TERM

Use these key terms to fill in the correct blank. Answers are at the end of the book.

adverse effect
controlled substance mark
DEA number
injunction
labeling

legend drug
liability
"look-alike" regulation
NDC (National Drug Code)
negligence

pediatric
placebo
recall
therapeutic

1. _____ : the number all prescribers of controlled substances are assigned and which must be used on all controlled drug prescriptions.

2. _____ : a court order preventing a specific action, such as the distribution of a potentially dangerous drug.

3. _____ : an inactive substance given in place of a medication.

4. _____ : an unintended side affect of a medication that is negative or in some way injurious to a patient's health.

5. _____ : any drug which requires a prescription and this "legend" on the label: Rx only.

6. _____ : failing to do something you should have done

7. _____ : having to do with the treatment of children.

8. _____ : important associated information that is not on the label of a drug product itself.

9. _____ : Federal laws require that a drug and/or its container not be imitative of another drug so that the consumer will be misled.

10. _____ : means you can be prosecuted for misconduct.

11. _____ : serving to cure or heal.

12. _____ : the action taken to remove a drug from the market and have it returned to the manufacturer.

13. _____ : the mark (CII-CV) which indicates the control category of a drug with a potential for abuse.

14. _____ : the number on a manufacturer's label indicating the manufacturer and product information.

TRUE/FALSE

Indicate whether the statement is true or false in the blank. Answers are at the end of the book.

_____ 1. Child-proof packaging was required by the Fair Packaging and Labeling Act.

_____ 2. Before it is approved for marketing, a new drug must be shown to be risk free.

_____ 3. Only about 25% of drugs tested on humans are approved for use by the FDA.

_____ 4. Over-the-counter medications do not require a prescription but sometimes prescriptions are written for them.

_____ 5. A prescription serial number must appear on the label of a dispensed prescription container.

_____ 6. Manufacturers are allowed to put controlled substance marks and storage requirements on accompanying labeling for their stock products rather than on the label itself.

_____ 7. Schedule II drugs must be stored in a locked tamper-proof narcotics cabinet.

_____ 8. Schedule III, IV, and V drugs may be stored openly on shelves in retail and hospital settings.

_____ 9. All controlled substances must be ordered using a DEA controlled substance order form.

_____ 10. Most recalls are voluntary.

EXPLAIN WHY

Explain why these statements are true or important. Check your answers in the text. Discuss any questions you may have with your Instructor.

1. Why is blind testing used in the drug approval process?

2. Give three reasons why OTC labels should be clear and understandable.

3. Why are some drugs "controlled" by the DEA?

4. Why are some drug patents extended past the original 17 year period.

5. Why would a manufacturer want to recall a drug product?

6. Give three reasons why failing to do something could result in a criminal charge of negligence.

MATCH THE TERM — CONTROLLED SUBSTANCES AND RECALLS

Use these key terms to fill in the correct blank. Answers are at the end of the book.

Schedule I Drugs   Schedule V Drugs
Schedule II Drugs   Class 1 Recall
Schedule III Drugs   Class 2 Recall
Schedule IV Drugs   Class 3 Recall

1. _____ :   Amphetamines, opium, cocaine, methadone, and various opiates are included on this schedule.

2. _____ :   Anabolic steroids and various compounds containing limited quantities of narcotic substances such as codeine are included on this schedule.

3. _____ :   When a product is not likely to cause adverse effects.

4. _____ :   Compounds containing limited amounts of a narcotic such as codeine are included in this group.

5. _____ :   When a product may cause temporary but reversible adverse effects, or in which there is little likelihood of serious adverse effects.

6. _____ :   Heroin, various opium derivatives, and hallucinogenic substances are included on this schedule.

7. _____ :   Phenobarbital, the sedative chloral hydrate, and the anesthetic methohexital are included in this group.

8. _____ :   When there is a strong likelihood that the product will cause serious adverse effects or death.

IDENTIFY

Identify the required elements on this manufacturer's bottle label by answering in the space beneath the question.

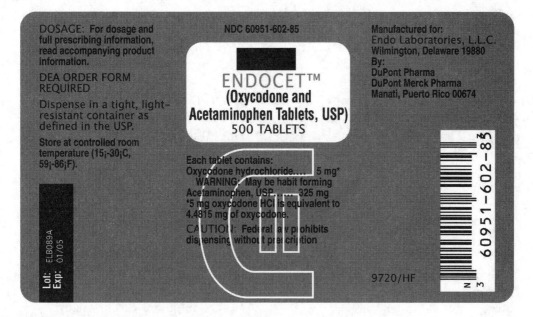

1. In what kind of container should this medication be dispensed?

2. Who is the manufacturer of this drug product?

3. What is the product's brand name?

4. What is the product's generic name?

5. What is the drug form?

6. What are the active ingredients?

7. What control level is the drug product?

8. What are the storage requirements?

9. What is the expiration date?

CHOOSE THE BEST ANSWER

Answers are at the end of the book.

1. The _____ defined what drugs require a prescription.
   a. 1970 Poison Prevention Packaging Act
   b. 1962 Kefauver-Harris Amendment
   c. Sherley Amendment
   d. 1951 Durham-Humphrey Amendment

2. A need for tighter drug regulations from the thalidomide lesson led to the
   a. Kefauver-Harris Amendment.
   b. Durham-Humphrey Amendment.
   c. Food and Drug Act of 1906.
   d. Food Drug and Cosmetic Act.

3. Legend drugs should have the legend _____ on the manufacturer's label.
   a. "Federal law prohibits transfer of this prescription"
   b. "Store at room temperature"
   c. "For external use only"
   d. "RX only"

4. In clinical trials, the testing is done
   a. on mice.
   b. on people.
   c. in vitro.
   d. on dogs.

5. The main purpose of phase I clinical trials is
   a. efficacy.
   b. dosage.
   c. safety.
   d. economics.

6. During clinical trials, a proposed new drug is called a(an)
   a. AZT.
   b. IND.
   c. CDRH.
   d. HMO.

7. The national drug code (NDC) is assigned by the
   a. FDA.
   b. DEA.
   c. CDER.
   d. manufacturer.

8. DEA form _____ is used to order Schedule II controlled substances.
   a. 007
   b. P19
   c. 222
   d. C41

9. In each state, pharmacists are licensed by the
   a. DEA.
   b. FDA.
   c. federal government.
   d. state board of pharmacy.

10. _____ means doing what is required.
    a. Compliance
    b. Negligence
    c. Insubordination
    d. Trafficking

Study Notes

Use this area to write important points you'd like to remember.

— 4 —

PHARMACEUTICAL TERMINOLOGY

KEY CONCEPTS

Test your knowledge by covering the information in the right hand column.

terminology	Much of medical science is made up of a small number of root words, suffixes and prefixes that originated from either Greek or Latin words.
root word	The base component of a term which gives it a meaning that may be modified by other components.
prefix	A modifying component of a term located before the other components of the term.
suffix	A modifying component of a term located after the other components of the term.
combining vowel	Combining vowels are used to connect the prefix, root, or suffix parts of the term.
cardiovascular system	Distributes blood throughout the body using blood vessels called arteries, capillaries, and veins.
endocrine system	Consists of the glands that secrete hormones (chemicals that assist in regulating body functions).
gastrointestinal (GI) tract	Contains the organs that are involved in the digestion of foods and the absorption of nutrients.
integumentary system	The body's first line of defense, acting as a barrier against disease and other hazards.
lymphatic system	The center of the body's immune system. Lymphocytes are a white blood cell that helps the body defend itself against bacteria and diseased cells.
muscular system	The body contains more than 600 muscles which give shape and movement to it.

nervous system	The body's system of communication. The neuron (nerve cell) is its basic functional unit.
skeletal system	Protects soft organs and provides structure and support for the body's organ systems.
female reproductive system	Produces hormones (estrogen, progesterone), controls menstruation, and provides for childbearing.
male reproductive system	Produces sperm and secretes the hormone testosterone.
respiratory system	Brings oxygen into the body through inhalation and expels carbon dioxide gas through exhalation.
urinary system	The primary organ is the kidney, which filters the blood for unwanted material and makes urine.
ear	The sense of hearing, as well as the maintenance of body equilibrium, is performed by the ear.
eyes	The eyelids protect the eye and assist in its lubrication. The conjunctiva is the blood-rich membrane between the eye and the eyelid.
drug classifications	A grouping of a number of drugs that have some properties in common. The same steps in interpreting other medical science terminology can be used to interpret drug classification names.

STUDY NOTES

Use this area to write important points you'd like to remember.

ORGAN SYSTEM ROOTS

CARDIOVASCULAR SYSTEM

angi	vessel
aort	aorta
card	heart
oxy	oxygen
pector	chest
phleb	vein
stenosis	narrowing
thromb	clot
vas(cu)	blood vessel
ven	vein

ENDOCRINE SYSTEM

lipid	fat
nephr	kidney
thym	thymus
adrena	adrenal
gluc	sugar
pancreat	pancreas
somat	body

GASTROINTESTINAL SYSTEM

chol	bile
col	colon
duoden	duodenum
enter	intestine
esophag	esophagus
gastr	stomach
hepat	liver
lapar	abdomen
pancreat	pancreas

INTEGUMENTARY SYSTEM

necr	death (cells, body)
derma	skin
cutane	skin
mast	breast
onych	nail

LYMPHATIC SYSTEM

aden	gland
cyt	cell
hemo, hemat	blood
lymph	lymph
splen	spleen

MUSCULAR SYSTEM

my	muscle
fibr	fiber
tendin	tendon

NERVOUS SYSTEM

cerebr	cerebrum
encephal	brain
mening	meninges
myel	spinal cord
neur	nerve

SKELETAL SYSTEM

arthr	joint
calcane	heel bone
carp	wrist
crani	cranium
dactyl	finger or toe
femor	thigh bone
fibul	small, outer lower leg bone
humer	humerus
myel	bone marrow, spinal cord
oste	bone
patell	kneecap
ped, pod	foot
pelv	pelvis
phalang	bones of fingers and toes
rachi	spinal cord, vertebrae
spondy	backbone, vertebrae
stern	sternum, breastbone
tibi	large lower leg bone
vertebr	backbone, vertebrae

ORGAN SYSTEM ROOTS

FEMALE REPRODUCTIVE SYSTEM

gynec	woman
hyster	uterus
lact	milk
mamm	breast
mast	breast
metr	uterus
ovari	ovary
salping	fallopian tube
toc	birth
uter	uterine

MALE REPRODUCTIVE SYSTEM

andr	male
balan	glans penis
orchid, test	testis, testicle
prostat	prostate gland
sperm	sperm
vas	vessel, duct
vesicul	seminal vescles

RESPIRATORY SYSTEM

aer	air
aero	gas
pneum	lung, air
pulmon	lung
pector	chest
nasal	nose
sinus	sinus
laryng	larynx
bronch	bronchus
ox	oxygen
capnia	carbon dioxide

URINARY SYSTEM

cyst	bladder
vesic	bladder
ren	kidney
nephr	kidney
uria	urine, urination

HEARING

ot	ear
cusis	hearing condition
acous	hearing
audi	hearing
salping	eustachian tube
tympan	eardrum
myring	eardrum
cerumin	wax-like, waxy

SIGHT

blephar	eyelid
cor	pupil
dacry, lacrim	tear, tear duct
corne, kerat	cornea
retin	retina
irid, iri	iris
bi, bin	two
opia	vision

STUDY NOTES

Use this area to write important points you'd like to remember.

COMMON PREFIXES

a	without		medi	middle
ambi	both		melan	black
an	without		meso	middle
ante	before		meta	beyond, after, changing
anti	against		micro	small
bi	two or both		mid	middle
brady	slow		mono	one
chlor	green		multi	many
circum	around		neo	new
cirrh	yellow		pan	all
con	with		para	alongside or abnormal
contra	against		peri	around
cyan	blue		polio	gray
dia	across or through		poly	many
dis	separate from or apart		post	after
dys	painful, difficult		pre	before
ec	away or out		pro	before
ecto	outside		pseudo	false
end	within		purpur	purple
epi	upon		quadri	four
erythr	red		re	again or back
eu	good or normal		retro	after
exo	outside		rube	red
heter	different		semi	half
hom	same		sub	below or under
hyper	above or excessive		super	above or excessive
hypo	below or deficient		supra	above or excessive
im	not		sym	with
immun	safe, protected		syn	with
in	not		tachy	fast
infra	below or under		trans	across, through
inter	between		tri	three
intra	within		ultra	beyond or excessive
is	equal		uni	one
leuk	white		xanth	yellow
macro	large		xer	dry

COMMON SUFFIXES

ac	pertaining to		oi	resembling
al	pertaining to		ole	small
algia	pain		oma	tumor
ar	pertaining to		opia	vision
ary	pertaining to		opsia	vision
asthenia	without strength		osis	abnormal condition
cele	pouching or hernia		osmia	smell
cyesis	pregnancy		ous	pertaining to
cynia	pain		paresis	partial paralysis
eal	pertaining to		pathy	disease
ectasis	expansion or dilation		penia	decrease
ectomy	removal		phagia	swallowing
emia	blood condition		phasia	speech
gram	record		philia	attraction for
graph	recording instrument		phobia	fear
graphy	recording process		plasia	formation
ia	condition of		plegia	paralysis, stroke
iasis	condition, formation of		rrhea	discharge
iatry	treatment		sclerosis	narrowing, constriction
ic	pertaining to		scope	examination instrument
icle	small		scopy	examination
ism	condition of		spasm	involuntary contraction
itis	inflammation		stasis	stop or stand
ium	tissue		tic	pertaining to
lith	stone, calculus		tocia	childbirth, labor
logy	study of		tomy	incision
malacia	softening		toxic	poison
megaly	enlargement		tropic	stimulate
meter	measuring instrument		ula	small
metry	measuring process		y	condition, process

COMMON MEDICAL ABBREVIATIONS

AAA	Abdominal aortic aneurysm		KVO	Keep vein open
ABG	Arterial blood gases		LBW	Low birth weight
ADD	Attention deficit disorder		LDL	Low density lipoprotein
AIDS	Acquired immunodeficiency syndrome		LKS	Liver, kidney, spleen
ALL	Acute lymphocytic leukemia		LOC	Loss of consciousness
AV	Atrial-ventricular		MG	Myasthenia gravis
AMI	Acute myocardial infarction		MI	Myocardial infarction
ANS	Autonomic nervous system		MICU	Medical intensive care unit
BM	Bowel movement		MRI	Magnetic resonance imaging
BP	Blood pressure		NKO	No known allergies
BPH	Benign prostatic hyperplasia		NPO	Nothing by mouth
BSA	Body surface area		NVD	Nausea, vomiting, diarrhea
CA	Cancer		OTC	Over the counter pharmaceuticals
CAD	Coronary artery disease		PAP	Pulmonary artery pressure
CF	Cardiac failure		PUD	Peptic ulcer disease
CHF	Congestive heart failure		PVD	Peripheral vascular disease
CMV	Cytomegalovirus		RA	Rheumatoid arthritis
CNS	Central nervous system		RBC	Red blood count or red blood cell
COPD	Chronic obstructive pulmonary diease		ROM	Range of motion
CV	Cardiovascular		s	Without
CVA	Cerebrovascular accident (stroke)		SaO2	Systemic arterial oxygen saturation
DI	Diabetes insipidus		SOB	Short of breath
DM	Diabetes melitus		STD	Sexually transmitted diseases
DOB	Date of birth		T	Temperature
DX	Diagnosis		T&C	Type and cross-match
ECG/EKG	Electrocardiogram		TAH	Total abdominal hysterectomy
ENT	Ears, nose, throat		TB	Tuberculosis
GERD	Gastroesophageal reflux disease		TPN	Total parenteral nutrition
GI	Gastrointestinal		Tx	Treatment
H	Hypodermic		U	Units
HA	Headache		U/A	Urinalysis
HBP	High blood pressure		UCHD	Usual childhood diseases
HDL	High density lipoprotein		URD	Upper respiratory diseases
HIV	Human immunodeficiency virus		UTI	Urinary tract infection
HR	Heart rate		VD	Venereal disease
ID	Infectious diseases		WBC	White blood count/cell
IH	Infectious hepatitis		WT	Weight
IO, I/O	Fluid intake and output		XX	Female sex chromosome
IOP	Intraocular pressure		XY	Male sex chromosome

FILL IN THE KEY TERM

Use these key terms to fill in the correct blank. Answers are at the end of the book.

anorexia	endocrine	hypothyroidism	sinusitis
arteriosclerosis	endometriosis	leukemia	somatic
bronchitis	gastritis	lymphoma	subcutaneous
cardiomyopathy	hematoma	neuralgia	tendinitis
colitis	hemophilia	osteoarthritis	thrombosis
conjunctivitis	hepatitis	phlebitis	transdermal
cystitis	hyperlipidemia	prostatitis	uremia
dermatitis	hypertension	pulmonary	vaginitis

1. _____ : high blood pressure.
2. _____ : condition of having blood clots in the vascular system.
3. _____ : inflammation of a vein.
4. _____ : hardening of the arteries.
5. _____ : disease of the heart muscle.
6. _____ : pertaining to the glands that secrete onto the bloodstream.
7. _____ : abnormally high amounts of fats in the blood.
8. _____ : a deficiency of thyroid secretion.
9. _____ : pertaining to the body.
10. _____ : loss of appetite.
11. _____ : inflamed or irritable colon.
12. _____ : inflammation of the liver from various causes.
13. _____ : inflammation of the stomach.
14. _____ : skin inflammation.
15. _____ : beneath the skin.
16. _____ : through the skin.
17. _____ : a collection of blood, often clotted.
18. _____ : a disease in which the blood does not clot normally.
19. _____ : lymphatic system tumor.
20. _____ : a disease of blood forming tissues.
21. _____ : inflammation of a tendon.
22. _____ : severe pain in a nerve.
23. _____ : chronic disease of bones and joints.
24. _____ : abnormal growth of uteral tissue within the pelvis.
25. _____ : inflammation of the vagina.
26. _____ : inflammation of prostate.
27. _____ : inflammation of bronchial membranes.
28. _____ : pertaining to the lungs.
29. _____ : inflammation of the sinuses.
30. _____ : inflammation of the bladder.
31. _____ : toxic blood condition caused by kidney disorders.
32. _____ : inflammation of the conjunctiva.

CHOOSE THE BEST ANSWER

Answers are at the end of the book.

1. The system of medical and pharmaceutical nomenclature is made of these four elements:
   a. prefixes, suffixes, root words, and combining vowels.
   b. prefixes, suffixes, key words, and combining vowels.
   c. prefixes, suffixes, key words, and combining consonants.
   d. prefixes, suffixes, root words, and combining consonants.

2. The root word "nephr" refers to the
   a. sinus.
   b. kidney.
   c. liver.
   d. body.

3. Hematemesis is the vomiting of
   a. partially digested food.
   b. the liver.
   c. blood.
   d. bile.

4. Fibromyalgia means
   a. brittle hair and nails.
   b. inflammation of a tendon.
   c. lymph node disease.
   d. chronic pain in the muscles.

5. Encephalitis means
   a. severe pain in a nerve.
   b. joint pain.
   c. inflammation of the brain.
   d. tumor of nerve cells.

6. Prostatitis means
   a. a prostate stone.
   b. inability to produce semen.
   c. inflammation of the testes.
   d. inflammation of the prostate.

7. The primary organ of the urinary tract is the
   a. liver.
   b. kidney.
   c. bladder.
   d. intestine.

8. Blepharitis means
   a. inflammation of the inside of the eye.
   b. inflammation of sinuses.
   c. inflammation of eyelids.
   d. inflammation of gums.

9. The suffix "megaly" means
   a. tissue.
   b. pain.
   c. enlargement.
   d. recording process.

10. The suffix "philia" means
    a. condition of.
    b. attraction for.
    c. fear of.
    d. pain.

STUDY NOTES

Use this area to write important points you'd like to remember.

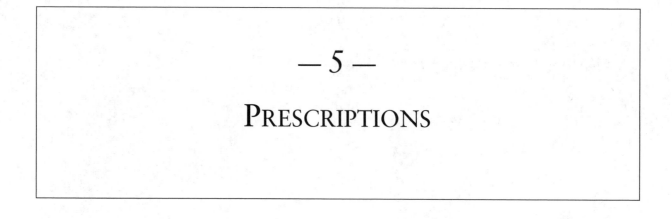

KEY CONCEPTS

Test your knowledge by covering the information in the right hand column.

prescription	A written order from a practitioner for the preparation and administration of a medicine or a device. Medical doctors (MD), dentists (DDS), veterinarians (DVM), and doctors of osteopathy (DO) are the primary practitioners allowed to write prescriptions. In some states, nurse practitioners, physicians assistants, and/or pharmacists are also allowed limited rights to prescribe medications.
medication orders	Used in institutional settings instead of a prescription form.
technician responsibilities	In community pharmacies, this generally includes receiving the prescription, collecting patient data, entering it into a computerized prescription system, and filling orders.
pharmacist role	Does all consulting with patients, handles Schedule II prescriptions, and checks all filled orders before dispensing.
prescription verification	It is necessary to check with the pharmacist on potential forgeries, on prescriptions that are more than a few days old, or on prescriptions that in any way appear questionable.
online billing	A prescription is interpreted and confirmed by the prescription system. If third party billing is involved, this is done online simultaneously.
preparation	Once the prescription and third-party billing is confirmed, the label and receipt are printed and the prescription is prepared.
label	The general purpose of the prescription label is to provide information to the patient regarding the dispensed medication and how to take it. Additionally, the label includes information about the pharmacy, the patient, the prescriber, and the prescription or transaction number assigned to the prescription.

signa	Directions for use. Since the patient is expected to self-administer the medication, these must be clear and easily understood by the patient.
pharmacist check	If a prescription has been prepared by a technician, there is a final check by the pharmacist to make sure that it is correct.
institutional settings	There are different requirements for institutional prescriptions since nursing staff generally administer medications to patients. Rules for institutional pharmacy prescription labels vary by institution but often do not contain much more than the name, strength, manufacturer, expiration date, and dosage form of the medication.
OTC prescriptions	Prescriptions may be written for over-the-counter (OTC) medications.
judgment questions	Technicians must request the advice of the pharmacist whenever judgment is required.
labels	Computer-generated prescription labels must be placed on containers so they are easy to locate and easy to read.
auxiliary labels	Many computerized prescription systems will automatically indicate which auxiliary labels to use with each drug.
controlled substance labels	Schedules II, III and IV substances must carry an auxiliary label stating: "Caution: Federal law prohibits the transfer of this drug to any person other than the patient for whom it was prescribed."

STUDY NOTES

Use this area to write important points you'd like to remember.

COMMON PHARMACY ABBREVIATIONS

Here are the most common pharmacy abbreviations.

ROUTE

a.d.	right ear
a.s., a.l.	left ear
a.u.	each ear
i.m., IM	intramuscular
inj.	injection
i.v., IV	intravenous
i.v.p., IVP	intravenous push
IVPB	intravenous piggyback
o.d.	right eye
o.s., o.l.	left eye
o.u.	each eye
per neb	by nebulizer
p.o.	by mouth
p.r.	rectally, into the rectum
p.v.	vaginally, into the vagina
SC, subc, subq	subcutaneously
S.L.	sublingually, under the tongue
top.	topically, locally

FORM

aq, aqua	water
caps	capsules
cm	cream
elix.	elixir
liq.	liquid
supp.	suppository
SR, XR, XL	slow/extended release
syr.	syrup
tab.	tablet
ung., oint.	ointment

TIME

a.c.	before food, before meals
a.m.	morning
b.i.d., bid	twice a day
h	hour, at the hour of
h.s.	at bedtime
p.c.	after food, after meals
p.m.	afternoon or evening
p.r.n., prn	as needed
q.i.d., qid	four times a day
q	each, every

q.d.	every day
q_h	every hour
qod	every other day
stat.	immediately
t.i.d., tid	three times a day

MEASUREMENT

$\bar{\text{i}}$	one
a.a. or aa	of each
ad	to, up to
aq. ad	add water up to
dil.	dilute
div.	divide
f, fl.	fluid
fl. oz.	fluid ounce
g., G., gm.	gram
gtt.	drop
l, L	liter/Litre
mcg.	microgram
mEq.	milliequivalent
mg.	milligram
ml., mL	milliliter/millilitre
q.s.	a sufficient quantity
q.s. ad	add sufficient quantity to make
$\bar{\bar{\text{ss}}}$	one-half
tbsp.	tablespoon
tsp.	teaspoon

OTHER

c	with
disp.	dispense
f, ft.	make, let it be made
gtt	drop
NR	no refill
$\bar{\text{s}}$	without
ut dict., u.d.	as directed
sig.	write, label

Note that the use of periods in abbreviations varies greatly. It is important to be able to recognize abbreviations with or without periods.

FILL IN THE BLANK

Answers are at the end of the book.

a.a. or aa	1. _____		l.	32. _____
a.c.	2. _____		liq.	33. _____
a.d.	3. _____		mcg.	34. _____
a.m.	4. _____		mEq.	35. _____
a.s.	5. _____		mg.	36. _____
a	6. _____		ml.	37. _____
a.u.	7. _____		NS	38. _____
ad	8. _____		o.d.	39. _____
aq	9. _____		o.s.	40. _____
aq. ad	10. _____		o.u.	41. _____
BSA	11. _____		p.c.	42. _____
bid	12. _____		p.o.	43. _____
c	13. _____		prn	44. _____
caps	14. _____		q	45. _____
per g button	15. _____		q.d.	46. _____
dil.	16. _____		q6h	47. _____
disp.	17. _____		qid	48. _____
per ngt	18. _____		q.s.	49. _____
D5W	19. _____		qsad	50. _____
elix.	20. _____		s̄	51. _____
f, fl.	21. _____		SC, s̈s̈	52. _____
g., G., gm.	22. _____		ss	53. _____
gtt.	23. _____		stat.	54. _____
h	24. _____		supp.	55. _____
h.s.	25. _____		syr.	56. _____
i.m., IM	26. _____		tid	57. _____
i.v., IV	27. _____		tab.	58. _____
i.v.p., IVP	28. _____		tbsp.	59. _____
NR	29. _____		top.	60. _____
IVPB	30. _____		tsp.	61. _____
L.	31. _____		ung.	62. _____
			u.d.	63. _____

THE PRESCRIPTION

Prescriber information:
Name, title, office address, and telephone number

Drug Enforcement Agency (DEA) registration number of prescriber
(required for all controlled substances)

Name and address of patient.
Other patient information such as age or weight is optional, but sometimes important, e.g., a child's weight.

Refill instructions

DAW
Dispense As Written and/or Generic Substitution Allowed instructions (optional).

Date the prescription is written.

Inscription: Name (brand or generic), strength of medication and quantity.

Signa: This comes from the latin word signa, meaning "to write." It is abbreviated to **sig** and indicates what directions for use should be printed on the label.

Signature of prescriber
(not required on a verbal prescription)

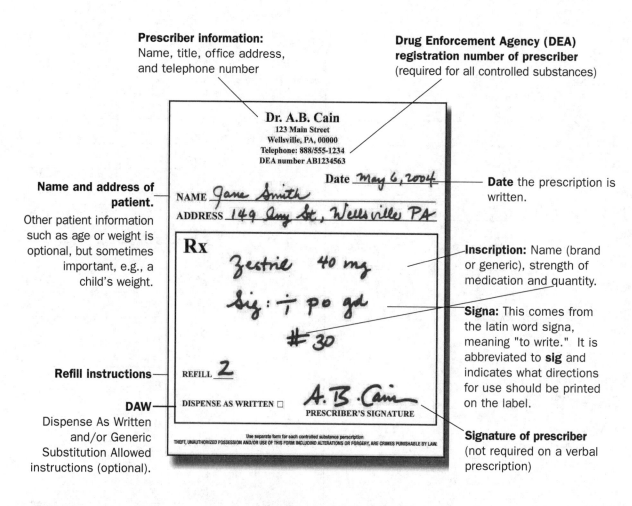

Note: If a compound is prescribed, a list of ingredients and directions for mixing is included.

Note: prescriptions are written in ink, never pencil.

PRESCRIPTION LABELS

the name, address, and telephone number of the pharmacy

the date dispensed

a prescription and/or transaction number

the name of the patient for whom the medication is dispensed

directions for use that are clear and accurate

the name, quantity, strength, manufacturer (name or NDC number), and dosage form of the medication dispensed

expiration date of the medication

the name of the prescriber

refill information.

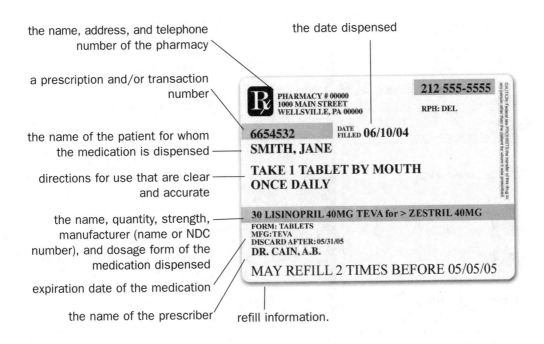

AUXILIARY LABELS

Additional, often colored auxiliary labels may also be applied to the prescription container in order to provide additional information to the patient (e.g. Shake Well, Keep Refrigerated, Take With Food or Milk). Many computerized prescription systems will automatically indicate which auxiliary labels to use.

Controlled substances from schedules II, III and IV must carry an auxiliary label stating:

Caution: Federal law prohibits the transfer of this drug to any person other than the patient for whom it was prescribed.

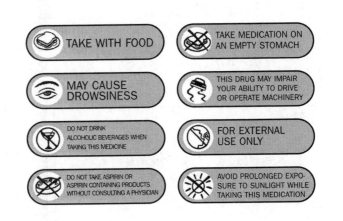

PRACTICE PRESCRIPTIONS

Identify the elements on these prescriptions by answering in the space beneath the question.

Dr. A.B. Cain
123 Main Street
Wellsville, PA, 00000
Telephone: 888/555-1234
DEA number AB1234563

Date *March 1, 2004*

NAME *D.H. Doe*

ADDRESS *345 Maple St, Wellsville PA*
D.O.B - 2/23/54

Rx

Prozac 20 mg

Sig: ÷ cap p.o. qd

#30

REFILL *X2*

DISPENSE AS WRITTEN ✓ *A.B.Cain*

PRESCRIBER'S SIGNATURE

Use separate form for each controlled substance perscription
THEFT, UNAUTHORIZED POSSESSION AND/OR USE OF THIS FORM INCLUDIND ALTERATIONS OR FORGERY, ARE CRIMES PUNISHABLE BY LAW.

1. What is the name of the drug?

2. What is the strength?

3. What is the dosage form?

4. What is the route of administration?

5. What is the dosage?

6. How many refills are there?

7. Can there be generic substitution?

JANE T. DOE, MD
1002 Main Street
WELLSVILLE, PA, 00000
(212) 555-5555

Date *6/5/04*

NAME *John Jones*

ADDRESS

Rx

Kenalog 0.1% Cream   15g
Apply BID

REFILL *1*

Doe

DEA No.

PRESCRIBER'S SIGNATURE

Use separate form for each controlled substance perscription
THEFT, UNAUTHORIZED POSSESSION AND/OR USE OF THIS FORM INCLUDIND ALTERATIONS OR FORGERY, ARE CRIMES PUNISHABLE BY LAW.

1. What is the strength of Kenalog Cream ordered by Dr. Doe?

2. How often should the medication be applied?

PRACTICE PRESCRIPTIONS

Identify the elements on these prescriptions by answering in the space beneath the question.

JANE T. DOE, MD
1002 Main Street
WELLSVILLE, PA, 00000
(212) 555-5555

Date _6/5/04_

NAME _Andrew Jones_

ADDRESS _____

Rx

Protonix 40 mg #60
T BID x 8 weeks

REFILL _1_

DEA No. _____

Doe

PRESCRIBER'S SIGNATURE

Use separate form for each controlled substance perscription
THEFT, UNAUTHORIZED POSSESSION AND/OR USE OF THIS FORM INCLUDIND ALTERATIONS OR FORGERY, ARE CRIMES PUNISHABLE BY LAW.

1. This prescription is written for Protonix. If the medication is taken as prescribed, every day, how many days will this prescription last?

2. How many refills have been ordered for this prescription?

JANE T. DOE, MD
1002 Main Street
WELLSVILLE, PA, 00000
(212) 555-5555

Date _6/5/04_

NAME _Steve Jones_

ADDRESS _____

Rx

Atrovent Inh #1 2-3 puff TID
Flovent 110 mcg #1 2 puff BID

REFILL _5_

DEA No. _____

Doe

PRESCRIBER'S SIGNATURE

Use separate form for each controlled substance perscription
THEFT, UNAUTHORIZED POSSESSION AND/OR USE OF THIS FORM INCLUDIND ALTERATIONS OR FORGERY, ARE CRIMES PUNISHABLE BY LAW.

1. By reading the box for the Atrovent Inhaler you find that each inhaler contains 200 inhalations. What is the days supply should be entered in the computer for the Atrovent prescription?

2. Flovent is dispensed in a 13 g canister that contains 120 metered doses. What is the days supply that should be entered in the computer for the Flovent prescription?

PRACTICE PRESCRIPTIONS

Identify the elements on these prescriptions by answering in the space beneath the question.

JANE T. DOE, MD
1002 Main Street
WELLSVILLE, PA, 00000
(212) 555-5555

Date __6/5/04__

NAME __Samuel Jones__

ADDRESS _____

Rx

Synthroid 0.05 mg *DAW* #30
T po qd

REFILL __5__

DEA No. _____

Doe

PRESCRIBER'S SIGNATURE

Use separate form for each controlled substance perscription
THEFT, UNAUTHORIZED POSSESSION AND/OR USE OF THIS FORM INCLUDIND ALTERATIONS OR FORGERY, ARE CRIMES PUNISHABLE BY LAW.

1. This patient has a dual co-pay of $15 for brand and $5 for generic. The patient has requested the generic for this prescription. What is written on the prescription that does not allow the generic to be dispensed?

JANE T. DOE, MD
1002 Main Street
WELLSVILLE, PA, 00000
(212) 555-5555

Date __6/5/04__

NAME __Francis Jones__

ADDRESS _____

Rx

Miacalcin 200 IU / inh
T inh qd (alt. nostrils)

REFILL __1__

DEA No. _____

Doe

PRESCRIBER'S SIGNATURE

Use separate form for each controlled substance perscription
THEFT, UNAUTHORIZED POSSESSION AND/OR USE OF THIS FORM INCLUDIND ALTERATIONS OR FORGERY, ARE CRIMES PUNISHABLE BY LAW.

1. How should the patient use this medication?

PRACTICE PRESCRIPTIONS

Identify the elements on these prescriptions by answering in the space beneath the question.

JANE T. DOE, MD
1002 Main Street
WELLSVILLE, PA, 00000
(212) 555-5555

Date _6/5/04_

NAME _Sandra Jones_

ADDRESS _____

Rx

Metrogel Vaginal 70 g
T applic PV qhs x 5D

REFILL _nr_

DEA No. _____

PRESCRIBER'S SIGNATURE _Doe_

Use separate form for each controlled substance perscription
THEFT, UNAUTHORIZED POSSESSION AND/OR USE OF THIS FORM INCLUDIND ALTERATIONS OR FORGERY, ARE CRIMES PUNISHABLE BY LAW.

1. What does 70 g mean for this prescription?

2. What does PV mean?

JANE T. DOE, MD
1002 Main Street
WELLSVILLE, PA, 00000
(212) 555-5555

Date _6/5/04_

NAME _Joyce Jones_

ADDRESS _____

Rx

Premarin 1.25 mg #21
T qd x 21, off 7

Provera 10 mg #5
1qd days 10-14

REFILL _5_

DEA No. _____

PRESCRIBER'S SIGNATURE _Doe_

Use separate form for each controlled substance perscription
THEFT, UNAUTHORIZED POSSESSION AND/OR USE OF THIS FORM INCLUDIND ALTERATIONS OR FORGERY, ARE CRIMES PUNISHABLE BY LAW.

1. How many days will the Premarin prescription last?

1. How many days will the Provera prescription last?

PRACTICE PRESCRIPTIONS

Identify the elements on these prescriptions by answering in the space beneath the question.

JANE T. DOE, MD
1002 Main Street
WELLSVILLE, PA, 00000
(212) 555-5555

Date __6/5/04__

NAME __Cindy Jones__

ADDRESS _____

Rx

Ortho-Novum 777 28 day
Ŧ QD

REFILL __6__

Doe

DEA No. _____

PRESCRIBER'S SIGNATURE

Use separate form for each controlled substance perscription
THEFT, UNAUTHORIZED POSSESSION AND/OR USE OF THIS FORM INCLUDIND ALTERATIONS OR FORGERY, ARE CRIMES PUNISHABLE BY LAW.

1. What is the total number of compacts indicated by this prescription (including the original fill plus refills)?

JANE T. DOE, MD
1002 Main Street
WELLSVILLE, PA, 00000
(212) 555-5555

Date __6/5/04__

NAME __Jane Jones__

ADDRESS _____

Rx

Bactrim DS 20
Ŧ po BID

REFILL __nr__

Doe

DEA No. _____

PRESCRIBER'S SIGNATURE

Use separate form for each controlled substance perscription
THEFT, UNAUTHORIZED POSSESSION AND/OR USE OF THIS FORM INCLUDIND ALTERATIONS OR FORGERY, ARE CRIMES PUNISHABLE BY LAW.

1. As you are entering this prescription in the computer, an allergy warning is displayed on the computer screen. What type of allergy does Jane Jones have?

PRACTICE PRESCRIPTIONS

Identify the elements on these prescriptions by answering in the space beneath the question.

JANE T. DOE, MD
1002 Main Street
WELLSVILLE, PA, 00000
(212) 555-5555

Date __6/5/04__

NAME __Ann Jones__

ADDRESS _____

Rx

Lorabid 200 mg/5 ml
iȝ po BID x 10

REFILL __nr__

Doe

DEA No. _____

PRESCRIBER'S SIGNATURE

Use separate form for each controlled substance perscription
THEFT, UNAUTHORIZED POSSESSION AND/OR USE OF THIS FORM INCLUDIND ALTERATIONS OR FORGERY, ARE CRIMES PUNISHABLE BY LAW.

1. What directions should be placed on the label for this prescription?

JANE T. DOE, MD
1002 Main Street
WELLSVILLE, PA, 00000
(212) 555-5555

Date __6/5/04__

NAME __Tom Jones__

ADDRESS _____

Rx

Amoxicillin 500 mg 2 po BID x 7
Biaxin 500 mg po BID x 7
Aciphex 20 mg po BID x 7

REFILL __nr__

Doe

DEA No. _____

PRESCRIBER'S SIGNATURE

Use separate form for each controlled substance perscription
THEFT, UNAUTHORIZED POSSESSION AND/OR USE OF THIS FORM INCLUDIND ALTERATIONS OR FORGERY, ARE CRIMES PUNISHABLE BY LAW.

1. How many capsules should be dispensed for the amoxicillin?

2. How many tablets should be dispensed for the Biaxin?

3. How many tablets should be dispensed for the Aciphex?

PRACTICE MEDICATION ORDERS

Identify the elements on this medication order by answering in the space beneath the question.

		DOCTOR'S ORDERS	PATIENT IDENTIFICATION
			099999999 675-01
			SMITH, JOHN
			12/06/1950
			DR. P. JOHNSON

DATE	TIME	DOCTOR'S ORDERS 1	DATE/TIME INITIALS	DATE/TIME INITIALS
1/3/04	22⁰⁰	Admit patient to 6ᵗʰ floor		
		Pneumonia, Dehydration		
		All: PCN- Rash		
		Order CBC, chem-7, blood cultures stat		
		NS @ 125ml/hr IV		
		Dr Johnson X2222		

DATE	TIME	DOCTOR'S ORDERS 2	DATE/TIME INITIALS	DATE/TIME INITIALS
2/01/04	3⁰⁰	Tylenol 650mg po q4-6 hrs PRN for Temp>38°C		
		Verbal Order Dr Johnson/ Jane Doe, RN		

DATE	TIME	DOCTOR'S ORDERS 3	DATE/TIME INITIALS	DATE/TIME INITIALS
2/01/04	6⁰⁰	Start Clarithromycin 500mg po q12°		
		Multivitamin po qd		
		Order CXR for this a.m.		
		Dr Johnson X2222		

1. What is the patient's disorder/condition?

2. Does the patient have allergies?

3. What route and dosage is ordered for the Tylenol 650mg?

4. What orders did the physician sign for?

5. What route and dosage are prescribed for the Clarithromycin?

6. What route and dosage are prescribed for the multivitamin?

7. What is the time span of these orders?

PRACTICE MEDICATION ORDERS

Identify the elements on this medication order by answering in the space beneath the question.

PATIENT:	John Smith		CITY HOSPITAL			
AGE:	35		PHYSICIAN'S ORDERS			
SEX:	m					
CHART #:	#123555					

				DIAGNOSIS:		
ALLERGIES:						

		ORDERS	SIGNATURE	COMPLETED OR DISCONTINUED		
DATE	TIME			NAME	DATE	TIME
		Meds:				
6/5/05	12:34 pm	① Lopressor 50 mg po qd				
		② HCTZ 25 mg po qd				
		③ Sonata 5 mg po hs prn				
		Doe				

PHARMACY COPY

1. What three medications have been ordered?

2. How often should the Sonata be taken?

53

PRACTICE MEDICATION ORDERS

Identify the elements on these medication orders by answering in the space beneath the question.

| PATIENT: *Mary Smith* | CITY HOSPITAL |
| AGE: SEX: CHART #: *35 F #123505* | PHYSICIAN'S ORDERS |

ALLERGIES: DIAGNOSIS:

COMPLETED OR DISCONTINUED

| DATE | TIME | ORDERS | SIGNATURE | NAME | DATE | TIME |

6/5/05 12:34pm Docusate Sod 100mg pro BID today

Start Metamucil tomorrow
ī tsp BID

Doe

PHARMACY COPY

1. What medication has been ordered for today?

2. What medication should be started tomorrow?

| PATIENT: *Andrew Smith* | CITY HOSPITAL |
| AGE: SEX: CHART #: *45 M 123616* | PHYSICIAN'S ORDERS |

ALLERGIES: DIAGNOSIS:

COMPLETED OR DISCONTINUED

| DATE | TIME | ORDERS | SIGNATURE | NAME | DATE | TIME |

6/5/05 10:22am Vit B12 1000 MCg IM Stat

Multivitamin ī po qd

Doe

PHARMACY COPY

1. What does STAT mean in the order for Vitamin B-12?

2. What is the route of administration for Vitamin B-12?

PRACTICE MEDICATION ORDERS

Identify the elements on these medication orders by answering in the space beneath the question.

PATIENT: Steve Smith	CITY HOSPITAL
AGE: 45	
SEX: m	PHYSICIAN'S ORDERS
CHART #: 123777	

ALLERGIES: Penicillin

DIAGNOSIS:

| DATE | TIME | ORDERS | SIGNATURE | COMPLETED OR DISCONTINUED NAME | DATE | TIME |

IVF NS @100 cc/hr x2 l

HCTZ 25 mg po qd

Diovan 80 mg po qd

Doe

PHARMACY COPY

1. What is the rate for the IV in this medication order?

2. What medications are to be given orally?

PATIENT: Barbara Smith	CITY HOSPITAL
AGE: 45	
SEX: F	PHYSICIAN'S ORDERS
CHART #: 123718	

ALLERGIES: Codeine

DIAGNOSIS:

| DATE | TIME | ORDERS | SIGNATURE | COMPLETED OR DISCONTINUED NAME | DATE | TIME |

6/3/04 10:00am FS AC + HS

Micronase 5mg po qd

Ambien 5mg po hs prn

Doe

PHARMACY COPY

1. What medications have been ordered?

2. Which medication would be administered at bedtime, as needed?

FILL IN THE KEY TERM

Use these key terms to fill in the correct blank. Answers are at the end of the book.

auxiliary label	institutional labels	protocols
DAW	lookalikes	Rx
DEA number	medication orders	Schedules II, III and IV auxiliary
extemporaneous compounding	prescription	label statement
inscription	prescription number	signa

1. _____ :   A written order from a practitioner for the preparation and administration of a medicine or a device

2. _____ :   The pharmaceutical preparation of a medication from ingredients.

3. _____ :   Specific guidelines for practice

4. _____ :   The directions for use on a prescription that should be printed on the label.

5. _____ :   The additional warning labels that are placed on filled prescription containers.

6. _____ :   The form used to prescribe medications for patients in institutional settings.

7. _____ :   Drug names that have similar appearance, particularly when written.

8. _____ :   Name (brand or generic), strength of medication and quantity.

9. _____ :   Dispense As Written, meaning generic substitution not allowed.

10. _____ :   An abbreviation of the latin word recipe, meaning "take."

11. _____ :   Often do not contain much more than the name, strength, manufacturer, expiration date, and dosage form of the medication.

12. _____ :   Caution: Federal law prohibits the transfer of this drug to any person other than the patient for whom it was prescribed.

13. _____ :   The number assigned to each prescription which appears on the label.

14. _____ :   Required on all controlled substance prescriptions.

TRUE/FALSE

Indicate whether the statement is true or false in the blank. Answers are at the end of the book.

_____ 1. In addition to the primary prescribers, nurse practitioners and physician assistants are allowed to write prescriptions in some states.

_____ 2. All prescriptions must be signed by the prescriber.

_____ 3. The signa indicates the medication and its strength.

_____ 4. If DAW is indicated, generic substitution may not be used.

_____ 5. A prescription has no time limit.

_____ 6. Patients with OTC prescriptions should be referred to the pharmacist.

_____ 7. One of the primary purposes of the prescription label is to provide the patient with clear instructions on how to take the medication.

_____ 8. Institutional labels must have the same information as in the community setting.

_____ 9. The prescription label may have either the date dispensed or the expiration date, but does not need both.

_____ 10. A DEA number is required on all prescriptions.

EXPLAIN WHY

Explain why these statements are true or important. Check your answers in the text. Discuss any questions you may have with your Instructor.

1. Why must the pharmacist always check the filled prescription before it is dispensed to the patient?

2. Why must the directions for use be clear and understandable to the patient in the community setting?

3. What are the differences between the prescription and the medication order? Why?

4. Why must prescriptions be written in ink?

5. Why are auxiliary labels important?

CHOOSE THE BEST ANSWER

Answers are at the end of the book.

1. Medication orders that are presented at community pharmacies are
   a. inscriptions.
   b. MARs.
   c. prescriptions.
   d. profiles.

2. In community pharmacies, _____ generally receive the prescription and collect patient data and enter this information into the computer.
   a. pharmacists
   b. pharmacy technicians

3. The _____ should be consulted on all OTC and Schedule II prescriptions.
   a. pharmacist
   b. pharmacy technician

4. When a prescription is written for a medication that is not commercially available, the medication can be prepared by mixing the ingredients required and this is called
   a. alligation.
   b. extemporaneous compounding.
   c. trituration.
   d. admixture.

5. If a new prescription has been prepared by a pharmacy technician, the final check is done by the
   a. lead pharmacy technician.
   b. pharmacist.
   c. patient.
   d. physician.

6. Prescriptions are written in
   a. ink.
   b. either ink or pencil.
   c. pencil.

7. The DEA Number is required on prescriptions for
   a. legend drugs
   b. medical devices
   c. controlled substances
   d. OTCs

8. The name of the drug, its strength, and quantity make-up the
   a. Insigna.
   b. Signa.
   c. Inscription.
   d. DAW Indicator.

9. Rx is an abbreviation of the Latin word recipe and means
   a. write.
   b. Sig.
   c. take.
   d. Insigna.

10. The route of administration should be indicated on the prescription if it is different from
    a. injectable
    b. rectal
    c. oral
    d. topical

11. When the Sig contains t.i.d., the medication should be taken _____ times a day.
    a. one
    b. two
    c. three
    d. four

12. Labels from _____ pharmacies contain more information than labels from _____ pharmacies.
    a. community, institutional
    b. institutional, hospital
    c. institutional, community
    d. hospital, institutional

CHOOSE THE BEST ANSWER

Answers are at the end of the book.

13. If a prescription requires extemporaneous compounding, the technician should inform the patient that
    a. the medication may be obtained without a prescription.
    b. there may be a delay in filling the prescription.
    c. a DEA number is required.
    d. any refills cannot be honored.

14. Medication Administration Records (MARs) in institutional settings are noted and signed by
    a. nurses
    b. doctors
    c. pharmacy technicians
    d. pharmacists

15. For the prescription: Amoxil 250 mg #30 i t.i.d. rfx2, how many days should the prescription last?
    a. 2
    b. 5
    c. 10
    d. 30

STUDY NOTES

Use this area to write important points you'd like to remember.

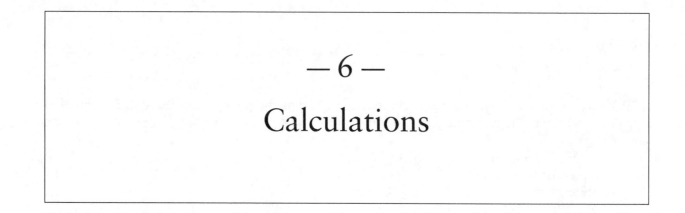

— 6 —

Calculations

RATIO AND PROPORTION

Most of the calculations pharmacy technicians will face on the job or in the certification exam can be performed using the *ratio and proportion* method.

A ratio states a relationship between two quantities. ➡ $\frac{a}{b}$

A proportion contains two equal ratios. ➡ $\frac{a}{b} = \frac{c}{d}$

When three of the four quantities in a proportion are known, the value of the fourth (x) can be easily solved. ➡ $\frac{x}{b} = \frac{c}{d}$

CONDITIONS FOR USING RATIO AND PROPORTION

1. Three of the four values must be known.

2. Numerators must have the same units.

3. Denominators must have the same units.

STEPS FOR SOLVING PROPORTION PROBLEMS

1. Define the variable and correct ratios.

2. Set-up the proportion equation

3. Establish the x equation

4. Solve for x.

5. Express solution in correct units.

Example

If there are 125 mg of a substance in a 500 ml solution, and 50 mg is desired, the amount of solution needed can be determined with this equation:

$$\frac{x \text{ ml}}{50 \text{ mg}} = \frac{500 \text{ ml}}{125 \text{ mg}}$$

multiplying both sides by 50 mg gives:

x ml = 2500 ml/125

solving for x gives:

x = 200

answer: 200 ml of solution are needed.

CONVERSIONS

Many proportion problems involve the use of conversions from one unit of measure to another. Here is a list of the most common.

Liquid Metric

1 L	=	10 dl	=	1000 ml
1 dl	=	0.1 L	=	100 ml
1 ml	=	0.001 L	=	0.01 dl

Solid Metric

1 kg	=	1,000 g		
1 g	=	0.001 kg	=	1,000 mg
1 mg	=	0.001 g	=	1,000 mcg
1 mcg	=	0.001 mg		

Avoirdupois

1 lb	=	16 oz
1 oz	=	437.5 gr
1 gr	=	64.8 mg (.0648 g)

Apothecary

1 gal	=	4 qt
1 qt	=	2 pt
1 pt	=	16 fl oz
1 fl oz	=	8 fl dr
1 fl dr	=	60 m

Household

1 tsp	=	5 ml		
1 tbs	=	3 tsp	=	15 ml
1 cup	=	8 fl oz		

Temperature

F temperature $= (1\frac{4}{5}$ times number of degrees C) + 32

C temperature $= \frac{5}{9}$ x (number of degrees F - 32)

$9C = 5F - 16$

Conversions Between Systems

1 L	=	33.8 fl oz		1 lb	=	453.59 g
1 pt	=	473.167 ml		1 oz	=	28.35 g
1 fl oz	=	29.57ml		1 g	=	15.43 gr
1 kg	=	2.2 lb		1 gr	=	64.8 mg

ROMAN NUMERALS

Roman numerals can be capital or lower case letters, and are:

ss = 1/2	L or l = 50
I or i = 1	C or c = 100
V or v = 5	D or d = 500
X or x = 10	M or m = 1000

RULES:

➡ When the second of two letters has a value equal to or smaller than that of the first, their values are to be added.

➡ When the second of two letters has a value greater than that of the first, the smaller is to be subtracted from the larger.

CONVERSION EXERCISES

Convert these numbers to decimals:

1. 1 1/4 _____
2. 0.5% _____
3. 6/8 _____
4. 2/3 _____
5. 8% _____
6. 42.5% _____
7. 3.2% _____

Write the following in Roman numerals:

15. 4 _____
16. 49 _____
17. 62 _____
18. 108 _____
19. 24 _____
20. 98 _____
21. 14 _____

Convert these numbers to percents:

8. .008 _____
9. 3/6 _____
10. 0.042 _____
11. 1/8 _____
12. 0.075 _____
13. 2/5 _____
14. 0.025 _____

Write the following in arabic numbers:

22. XXIV _____
23. CIV _____
24. MCC _____
25. iiss _____
26. XVIII _____
27. LIV _____

PROBLEMS

1. You have a prescription that calls for 1 cap po qid x 10 days. How many capsules are needed?

2. You have a prescription that calls for 1 cap po tid x 7 days. How many capsules are needed?

3. If a compounding order calls for Flagyl® 125 mg bid x 7 days, and only 0.5 gm tablets are available, how many tablets will it take to fill the order?

4. How much talc is needed for an order for 120 gm of the following compound: nupercainal ointment 4%, zinc oxide 20%, talc 2%?

5. A prescription calls for 200 mg of a drug that you have in a 10 mg/15 ml concentration. How many ml of the liquid do you need?

PEDIATRIC DOSES

Because of the many variables, conversion formulas for pediatric doses are rarely used in the pharmacy. Doses are generally given by the physician. **Children's doses are stated by kg of body weight (dose/kg).** Since 1 kg = 2.2 lb, you can solve for the prescribed dose by using a proportion equation if you know the child's body weight. See the following example.

An antibiotic IV is prescribed for an infant. The dose is to be 15 mg/kg twice a day. The baby weighs 12 lbs. How much drug is to be given for one dose? First the infant's weight in kilograms should be calculated.

x kg / 12 lb = 1 kg / 2.2 lb

$$\textbf{x} \text{ kg} = 12 \text{ lb times } \frac{1 \text{ kg}}{2.2 \text{ lb}} = \frac{12 \text{ kg}}{2.2} = 5.45 \text{ kg}$$

The next part of this problem can be solved with a simple equation.

one dose = 15 mg times 5.45 = 81.75 mg

PERCENTS & SOLUTIONS

Percents are used to indicate the amount or **concentration** of something in a solution. Concentrations are indicated in terms of weight to volume or volume to volume. The standard units are:

Weight to Volume: grams per 100 milliliters ➡ g/ml

Volume to Volume: milliliters per 100 milliliters ➡ ml/ml

A PERCENT SOLUTION FORMULA

Technicians find that they often have to convert a solution at one concentration to a solution having a different concentration, especially during the preparation of **hyperalimentation** or **TPNs.** It is possible to make such conversions using a simple proportion equation with these elements:

$$\frac{\textbf{x volume wanted}}{\textbf{want \%}} = \frac{\textbf{volume prescribed}}{\textbf{have \%}}$$

FLOW RATE

In some settings, the flow rate or rate of administration for an IV solution needs to be calculated. This is done using a ratio and proportion equation. Rates are generally calculated in ml/hour, but for pumps used to dispense IV fluids to a patient, the calculation may need to be done in ml/min or gtt/min.

For example, if you have an order for KCl 10 mEq and K Acetate 15 mEq in D5W 1000 ml to run at 80 ml/hour, you would determine the administration rate in ml/minute as follows:

x ml / 1 min = 80 ml / 60 min

x = 80/60 = 1.33

To get **drops per minute (gtt/min)**, you must have a conversion rate of drops per ml. For example, if the administration set for the above order delivered 30 drops per ml, you would find the drops per minute as follows:

$$\frac{80 \text{ ml}}{60 \text{ min}} \times \frac{30 \text{ gtt}}{1 \text{ ml}} = \frac{2400 \text{ gtt}}{60 \text{ min}} = 40 \text{ gtt/min}$$

MILLIEQUIVALENT—mEQ

Electrolytes are substances which conduct an electrical current and are found in the body's blood, tissue fluids, and cells. Salts are electrolytes and saline solutions are a commonly used electrolyte solution. The concentration of electrolytes in a volume of solution is measured in units called milliequivalents (mEq). They are expressed as milliequivalents per milliliter or equivalents per liter.

Milliequivalents are a unit of measurement specific to each electrolyte. For example, a 0.9% solution of one electrolyte will have a different mEq value than a 0.9% solution of another because mEq values are based on each electrolyte's atomic weight and electron properties, each of which is different.

If the mEq value of a solution is known, it is relatively easy to mix it with other solutions to get a different mEq volume ratio by using proportions.

EXAMPLE

A solution calls for 5 mEq of an electrolyte that you have in a 1.04 mEq / ml solution. How many ml of it do you need?

x ml/ 5 mEq = 1 ml/1.04 mEq

x ml = 5 ~~mEq~~ times $\frac{1 \text{ ml}}{1.04 \text{ mEq}}$ = $\frac{5 \text{ ml}}{1.04}$ = 4.8 ml

Answer: 4.8 ml of the solution is needed.

PROBLEMS

Use the preceding information to solve these problems

6. An IV requires the addition of 45 mEq potassium chloride (KCL). You have a vial of KCl at a concentration of 20 mEq per 10 ml. How many mls should be added?

7. If 360 grams of dextrose is ordered using a 50% dextrose solution, how many ml are needed?

8. A prescription calls for 0.36 mg of a drug that you have in 50 mcg/ml concentration. How many ml do you need?

9. The infusion rate of an IV is 300 ml over 4 hours. What is the ml/minute rate?

10. The infusion rate of an IV is 1000 ml over 12 hours. What is the rate per minute?

11. An IV order calls for administration of 1.5 ml/minute of a solution for four hours. How much solution will be needed.

12. If a physician orders 35% dextrose 1000 ml and all you have is 70% dextrose 1000 ml, how much 70% dextrose and how much sterile water will be used?

13. If a physician orders 20% dextrose 1000 ml and all you have is 70% dextrose 1000 ml, how much 70% dextrose and how much sterile water will be used?

14. If a physician orders 25% Dextrose 500 ml and you have 50% Dextrose 1000 ml, how much 50% Dextrose and how much sterile water do you need?

TOTAL PARENTERAL NUTRITION

A TPN order calls for the amounts on the left (including additives) to be made from the items on the right. The total volume is to be 1000 ml. How much of each ingredient and how much sterile water do you need to prepare this TPN ?

TPN Order	On Hand	
aminosyn 4.25%	aminosyn 8.5%	1000 ml
dextrose 20%	dextrose 50%	500 ml

Additives:

KCl	24 mEq	KCl 2mEq/ml	20 ml
MVI	5 ml	MVI	10 ml
NaCl	24 mEq	NaCl 4.4mEq/ml	20 ml

Figure out the amounts and enter the answer on the blank line.

1.) aminosyn _____

2.) dextrose _____

3.) KCl _____

4.) MVI _____

5.) NaCl _____

6.) sterile water _____

EXAMINATION NOTE: ALLIGATIONS

One type of problem that may appear on the certification exam specifies the use of the **alligation method** for mixing solutions of different concentrations. For example, how much of a 95% solution should be mixed with a 50% solution to create a 70% solution? Here's how to solve this using the alligation method.

a) Determine "**y**" (the amount needed of the weaker solution) by subtracting the desired solution concentration from the concentration with the highest percentage:
$$95\text{-}70 = 25$$

b) Determine "**x**" (the amount needed of the stronger solution) by subtracting the weaker solution concentration from the desired solution concentration:
$$70\text{-}50 = 20$$

c) The **x/y ratio is therefore 20/25**, with x indicating the number of parts of the higher percentage solution and y indicating the number of parts of the lower percentage solution needed for the mixture.

d) Interpret this as **20 parts of the 95% solution are needed for every 25 of the 50% solution.** (This can also be reduced to four parts of one for every five of the other.)

RETAIL MATH

Technicians in community pharmacies must know how to perform common retail calculations. Besides simple addition and subtraction, the most important calculations involve using percentages, especially in doing **mark-ups** or **discounts**. A mark-up is the amount of the retailer's **selling price minus their purchase cost**. It is calculated by multiplying the retailer's purchase cost by the mark-up percentage and adding the amount to the cost.

For example, a 30% mark-up on an item purchased for $2.30 is $0.69 (Note that 30% equals 0.3, and that $2.30 x 0.3 = $0.69), so the selling price would be $2.99 ($2.30 + $0.69).

Conversely, if you knew a $2.99 sale item was marked-up $0.69 and were asked to figure out the percent mark-up, you would subtract the $0.69 from $2.99 to get the cost of the item ($2.30), and then divide the mark-up by the cost: $0.69 ÷ $2.30 = 0.3 = 30%.

Discounts involve subtracting a percentage amount from the marked-up price of an item. A 30% discount on the $2.99 item is $0.90, so $2.09 would be the discounted price ($2.99-$0.90). Note that this is different than the cost of the item, because you deducted the percentage from the marked-up price.

— 7 —

ROUTES AND FORMULATIONS

KEY CONCEPTS

Test your knowledge by covering the information in the right hand column.

formulations

Drugs are contained in products called formulations. There are many drug formulations and many different routes to administer them.

route of administration

Routes are classified as enteral or parenteral. Enteral refers to anything involving the tract from the mouth to the rectum. There are three enteral routes: oral, sublingual, and rectal. Any route other than oral, sublingual, and rectal is considered a parenteral administration route. Oral administration is the most frequently used route of administration.

local and systemic effects

A local effect occurs when the drug activity is at the site of administration (e.g., eyes, ears, nose, skin). A systemic effect occurs when the drug is introduced into the circulatory system.

oral administration

The stomach has a pH around 1-2. Certain drugs cannot be taken orally because they are degraded or destroyed by stomach acid and intestinal enzymes. Drugs administered by liquid dosage forms generally reach the circulatory system faster than drugs formulated in solid dosage forms.

oral formulations

Oral formulations contain various ingredients beside the active drug. These inactive ingredients include binders, effervescent salts, lubricants, fillers, diluents, and disintegrants.

gastrointestinal action

The disintegration and dissolution of tablets, capsules, and powders generally begins in the stomach, but will continue to occur when the stomach empties into the intestine. Controlled-release or extended-release formulations extend dissolution over a period of hours and provide a longer duration of effect compared to plain tablets. Enteric coated tablets prevent the tablet from disintegrating until it reaches the higher pHs of the intestine.

sublingual administration	These tablets are placed under the tongue. They are generally fast dissolving uncoated tablets which contain highly water soluble drugs. When the drug is released from the tablet, it is quickly absorbed into the circulatory system since the membranes lining the mouth are very thin and there is a rich blood supply to the mouth.
rectal administration	Rectal administration may be used to achieve a variety of systemic effects, including: asthma control, antinausea, anti-motion sickness, and anti-infective. However, absorption from rectal administration is erratic and unpredictable. The most common rectal administration forms are suppositories, solutions, and ointments.
parenteral administration	Parenteral routes are often preferred when oral administration causes drug degradation or when a rapid drug response is desired, as in an emergency situation. The parenteral routes requiring a needle are intravenous, intramuscular, intradermal, and subcutaneous. These solutions must be sterile (bacteria-free), have an appropriate pH, and be limited in volume.
intravenous formulations	Intravenous dosage forms are administered directly into a vein (and the blood supply). Most solutions are aqueous (water based), but they may also have glycols, alcohols, or other non-aqueous solvents in them.
IV emulsions	Fat emulsions and TPN emulsions are used to provide triglycerides, fatty acids, and calories for patients who cannot absorb them from the gastrointestinal tract.
infusion	Infusion is the gradual intravenous injection of a volume of fluid into a patient.
intravenous sites	Several sites on the body are used to intravenously administer drugs: the veins of the antecubital area (in front of the elbow), the back of the hand, and some of the larger veins in the foot. On some occasions, a vein must be exposed by a surgical cut.
intramuscular injections	The principal sites of injection are the gluteal (buttocks), deltoid (upper arm), and vastus lateralis (thigh) muscles. Intramuscular injections generally result in lower but longer lasting blood concentrations than after intravenous administration.
subcutaneous injections	Injection sites include the back of the upper arm, the front of the thigh, the lower portion of the abdomen and the upper back. The subcutaneous (SC, SQ) route can be used for both short term and very long term therapies. Insulin is the most important drug routinely administered by this route.

KEY CONCEPTS

Test your knowledge by covering the information in the right hand column.

intradermal injections

Intradermal injections involve small volumes that are injected into the top layer of skin. The usual site for intradermal injections is the rear of the forearm.

ophthalmic formulations

Every ophthalmic product must be manufactured to be sterile in its final container. A major problem of ophthalmic administration is the immediate loss of a dose by natural spillage from the eye.

intranasal formulations

Intranasal formulations are primarily used for their decongestant activity on the nasal mucosa, the cellular lining of the nose. The drugs that are typically used are decongestants, antihistamines, and corticosteroids. Since nasal administration often causes amounts of the drug to be swallowed, in some cases this may lead to a systemic effect.

inhalations formulations

Inhalation dosage forms are intended to deliver drugs to the pulmonary system (lungs). Most of the inhalation dosage forms are aerosols that depend on the power of compressed or liquefied gas to expel the drug from the container. Gaseous or volatile anesthetics are the most important drugs administered via this route. Other drugs administered affect lung function, act as bronchodilators (bronchial tube decongestants), or treat allergic symptoms. Examples of drugs administered by this route are adrenocorticoid steroids (beclomethasone), bronchodilators (epinephrine, isoproterenol, metaproterenol, albuterol), and antiallergics (cromolyn).

dermal formulations

Most dermal dosage forms are used for local (topical) effects on or within the skin. Dermal formulations are used to treat minor skin infections, itching, burns, diaper rash, insect stings and bites, athlete's foot, corns, calluses, warts, dandruff, acne, psoriasis, and eczema. The major disadvantage of this route of administration is that the amount of drug that can be absorbed will be limited to about 2 mg/day.

vaginal administration

Formulations for this route of administration are: solutions, powders for solutions, ointments, creams, aerosol foams, suppositories, tablets, contraceptive sponges and IUDs. Vaginal administration leads to variable absorption since the vagina is a physiologically and anatomically dynamic organ with pH and absorption characteristics changing over time. Another disadvantage of this route is that administration of a formulation during menstruation could predispose the patient to Toxic Shock Syndrome.

TRUE/FALSE

Indicate whether the statement is true or false in the blank. Answers are at the end of the book.

_____ 1.   Sublingual administration is a parenteral route of administration.

_____ 2.   Oral administration is the most frequently used route of administration.

_____ 3.   With oral formulations, drugs administered by solid dosage forms generally reach the systemic circulation faster than liquid dosage forms.

_____ 4.   A low pH value such as 1 or 2 indicates a high acidity.

_____ 5.   Parenteral administration always involves the use of a needle.

_____ 6.   Emulsions are used in intravenous administration to deliver triglycerides, fatty acids and calories.

_____ 7.   Intramuscular injections generally cause more pain than intravenous injections.

_____ 8.   Insulin is routinely administered by the subcutaneous route.

_____ 9.   An advantage of ophthalmic administration is that most of the dose is always delivered to the eye.

_____ 10. Nasal formulations only have a local effect on the nasal mucosa.

EXPLAIN WHY

Explain why these statements are true or important. Check your answers in the text. Discuss any questions you may have with your Instructor.

1.   Give three reasons why a drug might not be used for oral administration.

2.   Give three reasons why a drug might not be used for parenteral administration.

3.   Why do most parenterals require skilled personnel to administer them?

4.   Why is the pH of intravenous solutions important?

5.   Why is the development of infusion pumps important?

6.   Why is it difficult to deliver drugs by inhalation?

FILL IN THE KEY TERM

Answers are at the end of the book.

adsorb	inspiration	solvent
aqueous	intradermal injections	sterile
atomizer	intramuscular injection sites	subcutaneous injection sites
biocompatibility	intravenous sites	sublingual administration
buccal cavity	IUD	systemic effect
colloids	lacrimal canalicula	topical
conjunctiva	lacrimal gland	Toxic Shock Syndrome
contraceptive	local effect	transcorneal transport
degradation	metered dose inhalers	transdermal patches
emulsions	nasal inhaler	trauma
enteric coated	nasal mucosa	viscosity
hemorrhoid	necrosis	water soluble
hydrates	parenteral	wheal
inactive ingredients	percutaneous	

1. _____ : When the drug activity is at the site of administration (e.g., eyes, ears, nose, skin).

2. _____ : When a drug is introduced into the circulatory system by any route of administration and carried to the site of activity.

3. _____ : The changing of a drug to a less effective or ineffective form.

4. _____ : The attachment of one chemical to another.

5. _____ : The pouch between the cheeks and teeth.

6. _____ : Ingredients beside the active drug that include binders, effervescent salts, lubricants, fillers, diluents, and disintegrants.

7. _____ : Coating that will not let the tablet disintegrate until it reaches the higher pHs of the intestine.

8. _____ : The property of a substance being able to dissolve in water.

9. _____ : When tablets are placed under the tongue

10. _____ : Painful swollen veins in the anal/rectal area.

11. _____ : Any route other than oral, sublingual, and rectal.

12. _____ : The death of cells.

13. _____ : Absence of all microorganisms, both harmful and harmless.

14. _____ : Injections administered into the top layer of the skin at a slight angle using short needles.

15. _____ : The veins of the antecubital area (in front of the elbow), the back of the hand, and some of the larger veins in the foot.

16. _____ : Water based.

17. _____ : A liquid that dissolves another substance in it.

18. _____ : An injury.

19. _____ : Particles up to a hundred times smaller than that those in suspensions that are, however, likewise suspended in a solution.

20. _____ : A mixture of two liquids that do not dissolve into each other in which one liquid is spread through the other by mixing and use of a stabilizer.

21. _____ : Gluteal (buttocks), deltoid (upper arm), and vastus lateralis (thigh) muscles.

22. _____ : The back of the upper arm, the front of the thigh, the lower portion of the abdomen and the upper back.

23. _____ : The thickness of a liquid.

24. _____ : Not irritating or infection or abscess causing to body tissue.

25. _____ : A raised blister-like area on the skin, as caused by an intradermal injection.

26. _____ : The gland that produces tears for the eye.

27. _____ : The tear ducts.

28. _____ : The eyelid lining.

29. _____ : Drug transfer into the eye.

30. _____ : The cellular lining of the nose.

31. _____ : Device used to convert liquid to a spray.

32. _____ : A device which contains a drug that is vaporized by inhalation.

33. _____ : Breathing in.

34. _____ : Aerosols that use special metering valves to deliver a fixed dose when the aerosol is activated.

35. _____ : The absorption of drugs through the skin, often for a systemic effect.

36. _____ : Applied for local effect, usually to the skin.

37. _____ : Absorbs water.

38. _____ : Deliver drugs through the skin for a systemic effect.

39. _____ : A rare and potentially fatal disease that results from a severe bacterial infection of the blood.

40. _____ : A device or formulation designed to prevent pregnancy.

41. _____ : An intrauterine contraceptive device that is placed in the uterus for a prolonged period of time.

IDENTIFY

Identify the route of administration.

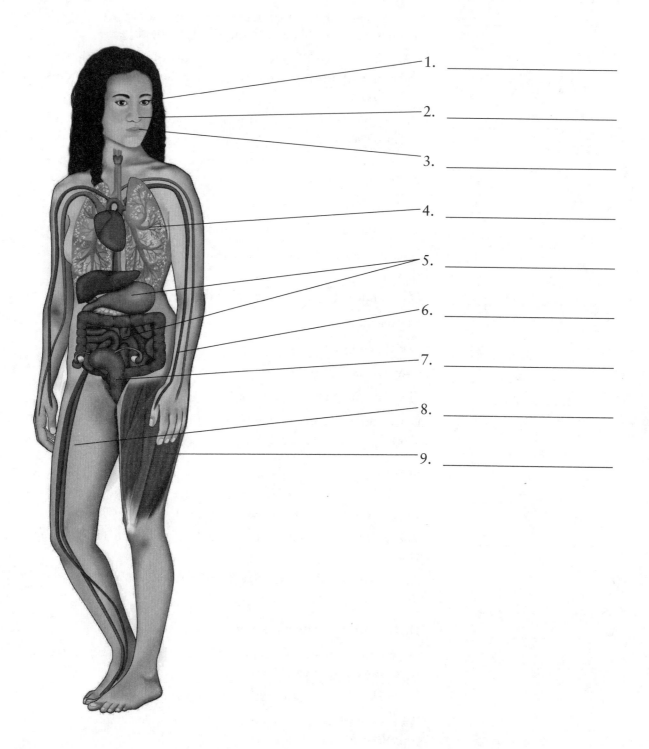

1. _____

2. _____

3. _____

4. _____

5. _____

6. _____

7. _____

8. _____

9. _____

IDENTIFY

Identify the routes of administration.

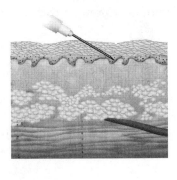

1. _____

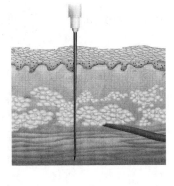

4. _____

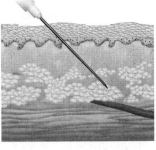

2. _____

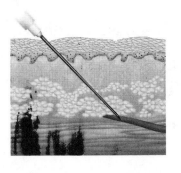

3. _____

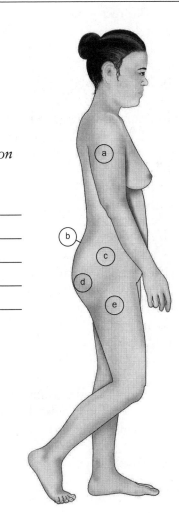

Identify these sites of intramuscular administration on the figure at right:

1. deltoid _____
2. gluteus maximus _____
3. gluteus medius _____
4. vastus lateralis _____
5. ventrogluteal _____

CHOOSE THE BEST ANSWER

Answers are at the end of the book.

1. _____ tablets are placed under the tongue.
   a. Enteric coated
   b. Buccal
   c. Sublingual
   d. TSS

2. _____ is the death of cells.
   a. Necrosis
   b. TSS
   c. Phlebitis
   d. Dermatitis

3. _____ injections are administered directly into veins.
   a. Subcutaneous
   b. Intravenous
   c. Transdermal
   d. Intramuscular

4. Inflammation of a vein is also known as _____ and can be a complication associated with intravenous administration.
   a. thrombus
   b. toxic shock
   c. phlebitis
   d. embolus

5. The gradual intravenous injection of a volume of fluid into a patient is called.
   a. transdermal
   b. infiltration.
   c. infusion.
   d. suspension.

6. The maximum amount of medication that can be administered subcutaneously is
   a. 0.5 ml.
   b. 2 ml.
   c. 0.2 ml.
   d. 5 ml.

7. The maximum volume for an intradermal injection is
   a. 2 ml.
   b. 1 ml.
   c. 5 ml.
   d. 0.1 ml.

8. The normal volume if tears in the eye is estimated to be
   a. 7 microliters.
   b. 2 ml.
   c. 5 ml.
   d. 3 ml.

9. The normal commercial eyedropper dispenses _____ of solution.
   a. 50 microliters
   b. 2 ml
   c. 1 ml
   d 0.5 ml

10. The most common size for an ophthalmic ointment tube is
    a. 10 g.
    b. 15 g.
    c. 3.5 g.
    d. 30 g.

11. MDIs are used to deliver drugs by
    a. inhalation.
    b. infusion.
    c. injection.

12. _____ absorption is the absorption of drugs through the skin, often for systemic effect.
    a. Intravenous
    b. Intramuscular
    c. Subcutaneous
    d. Percutaneous

13._____ are liquid preparation of pyroxylin dissolved in a solvent mixture of alcohol and ether.
a. Collodions
b. Emulsions
c. Elixirs
d. Suspensions

14._____ is an intrauterine contraceptive device that is placed in the uterus for a prolonged period of time.
a. Vaginal tablet
b. Vaginal sponge
c. TSS
d. IUD

STUDY NOTES

Use this area to write important points you'd like to remember.

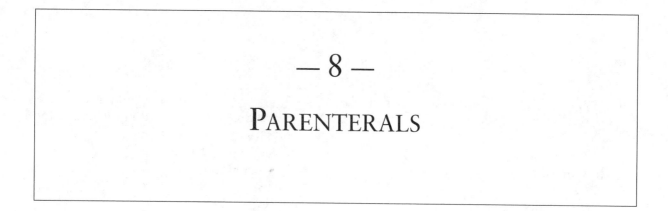

KEY CONCEPTS

Test your knowledge by covering the information in the right hand column.

parenteral solutions	There are two types of products: large volume parenteral (LVP) solutions and small volume parenteral (SVP) solutions. LVP solutions are typically bags or bottles containing larger volumes of intravenous solutions. SVP solutions are generally contained in ampules or vials.
properties	Solutions for injection or infusion must be sterile, free of visible particulate material, pyrogen-free, stable for their intended use, have a pH around 7.4, and in most (but not all) cases isotonic.
flow rate	The rate at which the solution is administered to the patient.
piggybacks	Small volumes of fluid (usually 50-100 ml) infused into the administration set of an LVP solution.
pumps	Infusion pumps, syringe pumps, and ambulatory pumps are devices used to administer LVP solutions and control flow rates. Administration sets are threaded through infusion pumps, and the pumps control the gravity flow. Infusion pumps have made the infusion process much more accurate and easier to administer and have been a major factor in the growth of home infusion.
admixtures	When a drug is added to a parenteral solution, the drug is referred to as the additive, and the final mixture is referred to as the admixture.
syringes	Syringes come in sizes ranging from 1 to 60 ml. As a rule, a syringe size is used that is one size larger than the volume to be measured. The volume of solution in a syringe is measured to the edge of the plunger's stopper while the syringe is held upright and all air has been removed from the syringe.
needle sizes	Needle sizes are indicated by length and gauge. The higher the gauge number, the smaller is the lumen (the hollow bore of the needle shaft). Large needles may be needed with highly viscous solutions but are more likely to cause coring.

filters	Often used to remove contaminating particles from solutions. Depth filters and membrane filters are the two basic groups.
laminar flow hood	Establishes and maintains an ultraclean work area for the preparation of IV admixtures.
aseptic techniques	Maintain the sterility of all sterile items and are used in preparing IV admixtures.
biological safety hoods	Used in the preparation of hazardous drugs. They protect both personnel and the environment from contamination.
percentage concentrations	Refer to the drug's weight per 100 ml if the drug is a solid, or the drug's volume per 100 ml if the drug is a liquid.
electrolyte solutions	Equivalent (Eq) or milliequivalent (mEq/l) are used to describe concentrations of electrolytes in solution.
parenteral nutrition solutions	These are complex admixtures composed of dextrose, fat, protein, electrolytes, vitamins, and trace elements. They are hypertonic solutions. Most of the volume of TPN solutions is made up of macronutrients: amino acid solution (a source of protein) and a dextrose solution (a source of carbohydrate calories). Several electrolytes, trace elements, and multiple vitamins (together referred to as micronutrients) may be added to the base solution to meet individual patient requirements. Common electrolyte additives include sodium chloride (or acetate), potassium chloride (or acetate), calcium gluconate, magnesium sulfate, and sodium (or potassium) phosphate. Multiple vitamin preparations containing both water-soluble and fat-soluble vitamins are usually added on a daily basis. A trace element product containing zinc, copper, manganese, selenium, and chromium may be added.
IV fat emulsions	Intravenous fat (lipid) emulsion is required as a source of essential fatty acids. It is also used as a concentrated source of calories. Fat provides nine calories per gram, compared to 3.4 calories per gram provided by dextrose. Intravenous fat emulsion may be admixed into the parenteral nutrition solution with amino acids and dextrose, or piggybacked into the administration line.
peritoneal dialysis solutions	Used by patients who do not have functioning kidneys to remove toxic substances, excess body waste, and serum electrolytes through osmosis. The solution is administered directly into the peritoneal cavity (the cavity between the abdominal lining and the internal organs) to remove toxic substances, excess body waste, and serum electrolytes through osmosis. These solutions are hypertonic to blood so the water will not move into the circulatory system.

LAMINAR FLOW AND BIOLOGICAL SAFETY HOODS

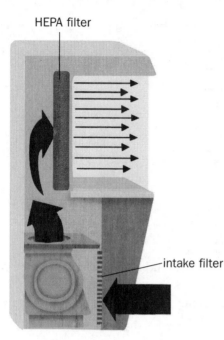

HEPA filter

intake filter

LAMINAR FLOW HOOD

With a Laminar flow hood, room air is drawn into a horizontal hood and passed through a prefilter to remove relatively large contaminants such as dust and lint. The air is then channeled through a high efficiency particulate air (HEPA) filter that removes particles larger than 0.3 µm (microns). The purified air then flows over the work surface in parallel lines at a uniform velocity (i.e., laminar flow). The constant flow of air from the hood prevents room air from entering the work area and removes contaminants introduced into the work area by material or personnel.

top down view

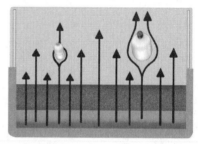

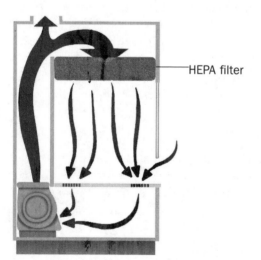

HEPA filter

BIOLOGICAL SAFETY HOOD

Biological safety hoods protect both personnel and the environment from contamination. It is used in the preparation of hazardous drugs. A biological safety cabinet functions by passing air through a HEPA filter and directing it down toward the work area. As the air approaches the work surface, it is pulled through vents at the front, back, and sides of the hood. A major portion of the air is recirculated back into the cabinet and a minor portion passes through a secondary HEPA filter and is exhausted into the room.

RULES FOR WORKING WITH FLOW AND SAFETY HOODS

✔ **Never sneeze, cough, talk directly into a hood.**

✔ **Close doors or windows.** Breezes can disrupt the air flow sufficiently to contaminate the work area.

✔ **Perform all work at least 6 inches inside the hood** to derive the benefits of the laminar air flow. Laminar flow air begins to mix with outside air near the edge of the hood.

✔ **Maintain a direct, open path between the filter and the area inside the hood.**

✔ **Place nonsterile objects, such as solution containers or your hands, downstream from sterile ones.** Particles blown off these objects can contaminate anything downstream from them.

✔ **Do not put large objects at the back of the work area next to the filter.** They will disrupt air flow.

ASEPTIC TECHNIQUE

HAND WASHING

✔ Remove all jewelry and scrub hands and arms to the elbows with a suitable antibacterial agent.

✔ Stand far enough away from the sink so clothing does not come in contact with it.

✔ Turn on water. Wet hands and forearms thoroughly. Keep hands pointed downward.

✔ Scrub hands vigorously with an antibacterial soap.

✔ Work soap under fingernails by rubbing them against the palm of the other hand.

✔ Interlace the fingers and scrub the spaces between the fingers.

✔ Wash wrists and arms up to the elbows.

✔ Thoroughly rinse the soap from hands and arms.

✔ Dry hands and forearms thoroughly using a nonshedding paper towel.

✔ Use a dry paper towel to turn off the water faucet.

✔ After hands are washed, avoid touching clothes, face, hair, or any other potentially contaminated object in the area.

CLOTHING AND BARRIERS

✔ Wear clean lint-free garments or barrier clothing, including gowns, hair covers, and a mask.

✔ Wear sterile gloves.

✔ Follow facility or manufacturer guidelines for putting on and removing barrier clothing. Unless barriers are put on properly, they can easily become contaminated.

TRUE/FALSE

Indicate whether the statement is true or false in the blank. Answers are at the end of the book.

_____ 1.   Pyrogens are a micronutrient in parenteral solutions.

_____ 2.   0.9% sodium chloride is an isotonic solution.

_____ 3.   Physiological pH is about 7.4.

_____ 4.   To practice aseptic technique, you must first sterilize your hands.

_____ 5.   Fat provides 9 calories per gram, compared to 3.4 calories per gram provided by dextrose.

_____ 6.   5% dextrose is used as an irrigation solution.

EXPLAIN WHY

Explain why these statements are true or important. Check your answers in the text. Discuss any questions you may have with your Instructor.

1.   Why should intravenous solutions generally be isotonic?

2.   Why is the position of objects on a laminar flow hood work surface important?

3.   Why is visual inspection of parenteral solutions important?

IN THE WORKPLACE

Use these tools to practice and check some of your workplace skills.

Pharmacy Technician Skills Checklist
ASEPTIC TECHNIQUE: HAND WASHING

Name: _____

Skill or Procedure	Self-Assessment		Supervisor Review		
	Needs to Improve	Meets or Exceeds	Needs to Improve*	Meets or Exceeds	*Plan of Action
1. Removes all jewelry and scrubs hands and arms to the elbows with suitable antibacterial agent.					
2. Stands far enough away from sink so clothing does not come in contact with sink.					
3. Turns on water, wets hands and forearms thoroughly, keeps hands pointed downward.					
4. Scrubs hands vigorously with antibacterial soap.					
5. Works soap under fingernails by rubbing them against the palm of the other hand.					
6. Interlaces fingers and scrubs the spaces between the fingers.					
7. Washes wrists and arms up to the elbows.					
8. Thoroughly rinses the soap from hands and arms.					
9. Dries hands and forearms thoroughly using a nonshedding paper towel.					
10. Uses a dry paper towel to turn off water faucet.					

Pharmacy Technician Skills Checklist
LAMINAR FLOW HOOD

Name: _____

Skill or Procedure	Self-Assessment		Supervisor Review		
	Needs to Improve	Meets or Exceeds	Needs to Improve*	Meets or Exceeds	*Plan of Action
1. Turns on and lets run for at least 30 minutes prior to use.					
2. Does not allow jewelry, long sleeves, or other non-sterile materials within the hood.					
3. Uses clean gauze/sponge to clean hood with 70% isopropyl alcohol.					
4. Uses long side-to-side motions on the back surface of the hood and works from top to bottom to clean hood.					
5. Uses back-to-front motions, working from the top to the bottom of each side to clean the sides of the hood.					
6. Uses back-to-front motions to clean the surface of the hood.					
7. Takes care so that cleaned surfaces do not become contaminated during cleaning.					
8. Takes care when placing items in hood so that airflow is not blocked.					
9. Takes care when preparing admixtures, that airflow is not blocked by hands or other objects.					
10. Takes care so that hands remain under the hood during admixture preparation, and does not leave the hood during admixture preparation.					
11. Does not utilize outer 6 inches of hood opening or work too closely to sides and back of hood during drug preparation and manipulations.					
12. Does not contaminate hood by coughing, sneezing, chewing gum, or excessive talking.					

IN THE WORKPLACE

Use these tools to practice and check some of your workplace skills.

Pharmacy Technician Skills Checklist
GLASS AMPULES

Name: _____

Skill or Procedure	Self-Assessment		Supervisor Review		
	Needs to Improve	Meets or Exceeds	Needs to Improve*	Meets or Exceeds	*Plan of Action
1. If ampule is not pre-scored, uses a fine file to lightly score the neck of the ampule at its narrowest point.					
2. Holds ampule upright and taps the top.					
3. Swabs neck of ampule with an alcohol swab.					
4. Wraps gauze pad around neck of ampule and quickly snaps ampule moving hands outward and away.					
5. Inspects opened ampule for glass particles.					
6. Tilts ampule (about 20 degree angle).					
7. Inserts needle into ampule, so needle point does not touch opening of ampule.					
8. Positions needle into solution placing beveled edge against side of ampule.					
9. Withdraws correct amount of the drug while keeping the needle submerged.					
10. Withdraws needle from ampule and removes air bubbles from syringe					
11. Transfers solution to final container using filter needle or membrane filter.					

Pharmacy Technician Skills Checklist
VIAL WITH SOLUTION

Name: _____

Skill or Procedure	Self-Assessment		Supervisor Review		
	Needs to Improve	Meets or Exceeds	Needs to Improve*	Meets or Exceeds	*Plan of Action
1. Takes care in removing vial cover.					
2. Uses care in cleaning top of vial with alcohol wipe.					
3. Draws into syringe a volume of air equal to the volume of drug to be withdrawn.					
4. Penetrates the vial without coring and injects air.					
5. Turns the vial upside down and withdraws correct amount of drug into syringe.					
6. Withdraws needle from vial and with needle end up, taps syringe to allow air bubbles to come to the top of the syringe. Presses plunger to remove air and excess solution.					
7. Transfers solution into the IV bag or bottle, minimizing coring.					

IN THE WORPLACE

Use these tools to practice and check some of your workplace skills.

Pharmacy Technician Skills Checklist
VIAL WITH POWDER

Name: _____

Skill or Procedure	Self-Assessment		Supervisor Review		
	Needs to Improve	Meets or Exceeds	Needs to Improve*	Meets or Exceeds	*Plan of Action
1. Takes care in removing vial cover.					
2. Uses care in cleaning top of vial with alcohol wipe.					
3. Draws into syringe a volume of air equal to the volume of diluent to be withdrawn.					
4. Penetrates the diluent vial without coring and injects air.					
5. Turns the diluent vial upside down and withdraws correct amount of diluent into syringe.					
6. Injects diluent into medication vial, and then withdraws a slight amount of air.					
7. Shakes vial until drug dissolves (unless shaking is not recommended)					
8. Reinserts needle and removes proper volume of drug solution (without injecting air).					
9. Removes all bubbles from syringe and transfers reconstituted solution to final container.					

Name: _____

Pharmacy Technician Skills Checklist
ADDING A DRUG (SVP) TO AN LVP

Skill or Procedure	Self-Assessment		Supervisor Review		
	Needs to Improve	Meets or Exceeds	Needs to Improve*	Meets or Exceeds	*Plan of Action
1. Removes protective covering from LVP package.					
2. Assembles the needle and syringe.					
3. If drug is in powder form, reconstitutes drug with recommended diluent.					
4. Swabs the SVP with an alcohol swab and draws the necessary volume of drug solution.					
5. Swabs the medication port of the LVP with an alcohol swab.					
6. Inserts needle into the medication port and through the inner diaphragm (medication port is fully extended).					
7. Injects the SVP solution.					
8. Removes the needle.					
9. Shakes and inspects the admixture					

FILL IN THE KEY TERM

Answers are at the end of the book.

admixture	dialysis	hypotonic	molecular weight
ampules	diluent	infusion	osmotic pressure
anhydrous	equivalent weight	ion	osmosis
aseptic techniques	final filter	irrigation solution	piggybacks
bevel	flow rate	isotonic	pyrogens
biological safety hoods	gauge	laminar flow	ready-to-mix systems
coring	HEPA filter	lumen	sharps
coring	heparin lock	lyophilized	valence
depth filter	hypertonic	membrane filter	waters of hydration

1. _____ : Techniques that maintain sterile condition.

2. _____ : Chemicals produced by microorganisms that can cause pyretic (fever) reactions in patients.

3. _____ : A characteristic of a solution determined by the number of dissolved particles in it.

4. _____ : When a solution has an osmolarity equivalent to another.

5. _____ : When a solution has a greater osmolarity than another.

6. _____ : When a solution has a lesser osmolarity than another.

7. _____ : The rate (in ml/hour or ml/minute) at which the solution is administered to the patient.

8. _____ : An injection device which uses heparin to keep blood from clotting in the device.

9. _____ : Small volume solutions added to an LVP.

10. _____ : The slow continuous introduction of a solution into the blood stream.

11. _____ : The resulting solution when a drug is added to a parenteral solution.

12. _____ : Freeze-dried.

13. _____ : A liquid that dilutes a substance or solution.

14. _____ : Systems with predetermined amounts of admixture components for which admixing takes place just prior to administration.

15. _____ : An angled surface, as with the tip of a needle.

16. _____ : With needles, the higher the number, the thinner the lumen.

17. _____ : The hollow center of a needle.

18. _____ : When a needle damages the rubber closure of a parenteral container, causing fragments of the closure to fall into the container and contaminate its contents.

19. _____ : A filter that attaches to a syringe and filters solution through a membrane as the solution is expelled from the syringe.

20. _____ : A filter placed inside a needle hub that can filter solutions being drawn in or expelled, but not both.

21. _____ : A filter that filters solution immediately before it enters a patient's vein.

22. _____ : Continuous movement at a stable rate in one direction.

23. _____ : A high efficiency particulate air filter.

24. _____ : Are used in the preparation of hazardous drugs and protect both personnel and the environment from contamination.

25. _____ : Large splash solutions used during surgical or urologic procedures to bathe and moisten body tissue.

26. _____ : Sealed glass containers with an elongated neck that must be snapped off.

27. _____ : Needles, jagged glass or metal objects, or any items that might puncture or cut the skin.

28. _____ : A drug's molecular weight divided by its valence, a common measure of electrolytes.

29. _____ : The number of positive or negative charges on an ion.

30. _____ : The sum of the atomic weights of one molecule.

31. _____ : Molecular particles that carry electric charges.

32. _____ : Without water molecules.

33. _____ : Water molecules that attach to drug molecules.

34. _____ : The action in which drug in a higher concentration solution passes through a permeable membrane to a lower concentration solution.

35. _____ : Movement of particles in a solution through permeable membranes.

CHOOSE THE BEST ANSWER

Answers are at the end of the book.

1. Pyrogens are chemicals that are produced by
   a. coring.
   b. microorganisms.
   c. precipitation.
   d. heat.

2. A(an) _____ solution has greater osmolarity than blood.
   a. hypotonic
   b. isotonic
   c. hypertonic
   d. pyrogenic

3. Piggybacks usually contain _____ of fluid and are infused over a period of 30-60 minutes.
   a. 50 - 100 ml
   b. 250 - 500 ml
   c. 5000 - 1000 ml
   d. 1000 ml - 2000 ml

4. When a drug is added to a parenteral solution, the drug is referred to as the _____ and the final mixture is referred to as the _____.
   a. admixture, additive
   b. suspension, solution
   c. additive, admixture
   d. solution, suspension

5. Some examples of ready-to-mix systems include
   a. heparin lock and Ringer's solution.
   b. Luer-Lok® and Slip-Lok®.
   c. Add-Vantage®, Add-a-Vial®, and Mini-Bag Plus®.
   d. Ringer's solution and Lactated Ringer's solution.

6. _____ is the term for fragments of a vial closure that contaminate a parenteral solution.
   a. Lumen
   b. Bevel
   c. Coring
   d. Hub

7. _____ are filters that can be placed inside of needles.
   a. Membrane filters
   b. Filter needles
   c. HEPA filters
   d. Intake filters

8. In horizontal laminar flow hoods, air blows
   a. down toward the work area.
   b. away from the operator.
   c. toward the operator.
   d. up toward the HEPA filter.

9. Biological Safety Hoods have
   a. vertical air flow down toward the work.
   b. horizontal air flow away from the operator.
   c. vertical air flow up toward the HEPA filter.
   d. horizontal air flow toward the operator.

10. When positioning supplies for use in a laminar flow hood
    a. larger supplies should be placed closer to the HEPA filter.
    b. smaller supplies should be placed closer to the HEPA filter.
    c. space the supplies close together to minimize laminar flow.
    d. the spacing of supplies has no effect on laminar flow.

11. Extemporaneous compounding refers to
    a. preparing an admixture for a specific prescription.
    b. LVPs that are commercially available and the compounding was completed by a pharmaceutical manufacturer.
    c. preparing admixtures in advance for commonly used prescriptions.
    d. SVPs that are commercially available and the compounding was completed by a pharmaceutical manufacturer.

12. If an ampule has not been pre-scored, the technician should
    a. score the neck of the ampule with a fine file.
    b. use sterile pliers to open the ampule.
    c. use a file to file all the way through the neck.
    d. just snap the ampule since manufacturers always pre-score when necessary.

13. Equivalent weight is equal to
    a. valence divided by molecular weight
    b. molecular weight divided by valence and multiplied by 2
    c. valence divided by molecular weight and multiplied by 2
    d. molecular weight divided by valence

14. Percent concentration for a solid ingredient equals
    a. weight in mg per 100 ml of solution.
    b. weight in g per 100 ml of solution.
    c. volume in ml per 100 ml of solution.
    d. weight in g per ml of solution.

15. Total parenteral solutions are
    a. dialysis solutions.
    b. hypotonic solutions.
    c. hypertonic solutions.
    d. isotonic solutions.

16. The movement of particles in a solution through permeable membranes is
    a. osmosis.
    b. pyrogenic.
    c. dialysis.
    d. HEPA.

STUDY NOTES

Use this area to write important points you'd like to remember.

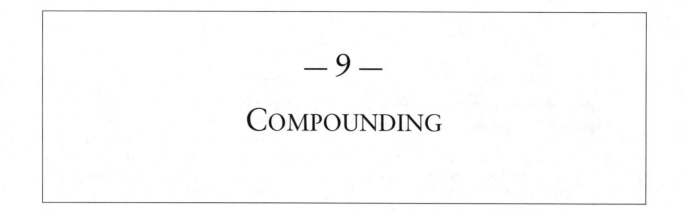

— 9 —

COMPOUNDING

KEY CONCEPTS

Test your knowledge by covering the information in the right hand column.

extemporaneous compounding	The on-demand preparation of a drug product according to a physician's prescription, formula, or recipe.
accuracy and stability	The supervising pharmacist must determine that a product can be accurately compounded and will be stable for its expected use. Accuracy is then essential in all weighings, measurements, and other activities in the compounding process.
class A balances	Can weigh as little as 120 mg of material with a 5% error. Always use the balance on a level surface and in a draft-free area. Always arrest the balance before adding or removing weight from either pan, or storing.
electronic or analytical balances	Highly sensitive balances that can weigh quantities smaller than 120 mg with acceptable accuracy.
weighing papers or boats	Should always be placed on the balance pans before any weighing is done. Balances must be readjusted after a new weighing paper or boat has been placed on each pan. Weighing papers taken from the same box can vary in weight by as much as 65 mg.
mortar and pestle	Made of three types of materials: glass, wedgwood and porcelain. Wedgwood and porcelain mortars are used to grind crystals and large particles into fine powders. Glass mortars and pestles are preferable for mixing liquids and semi solid dosage forms.
volumetric glassware	For weighing liquid drugs, solvents, or additives. Includes graduates, flasks, pipets and syringes. Erlenmeyer flasks, beakers, and prescription bottles, regardless of markings, are not volumetric glassware.
small volumes	Always use the smallest device (graduate, pipet, syringe) that will accommodate the desired volume of liquid.

graduated cylinders	Cylindrical graduates are preferred over cone shaped because they are more accurate. When selecting a graduate, always choose the smallest graduate capable of containing the volume to be measured. Avoid measurements of volumes that are below 20 percent of the capacity of the graduate because the accuracy is unacceptable.
disposable syringe	Used to measure small volumes. Measurements made with syringes are more accurate and precise than those made with cylindrical graduates. Measure volumes to the edge of the syringe stopper.
meniscus	The curved surface of a volume of liquid. When reading a volume of a liquid against a graduation mark, hold the graduate so the meniscus is at eye level and read the mark at the bottom of the meniscus.
medicine droppers	Used to deliver small liquid doses, but must first be calibrated.
trituration	The fine grinding of a powder.
levigation	The trituration of a powdered drug with a solvent in which the drug is insoluble to reduce the particle size of the drug.
geometric dilution	A technique for mixing two powders of unequal size. The smaller amount of powder is diluted in steps by additions of the larger amount of powder.
solvents	Water is the most common solvent, but ethanol, glycerin, propylene glycol, or a variety of syrups may be used.
sensitivity requirement	The amount of weight that will move the balance pointer one division mark.
nonaqueous solutions	Solutions that contain solvents other than water.
syrup	A concentrated or nearly saturated solution of sucrose in water. Syrups containing flavoring agents are known as flavoring syrups (e.g. Cherry Syrup, Acacia Syrup, etc.).
thickening agents	Reduce the settling (sedimentation rate) of a suspension.
suspensions	A "two-phase" compound consisting of a finely divided solid dispersed in a liquid. Most solid drugs are levigated in a mortar to reduce the particle size as much as possible before adding to the vehicle. Common levigating agents are alcohol or glycerin.
flocculating agents	Electrolytes that carry an electrical charge and enhance particle "dispersability" in a solution.
ointments and creams	Ointments are simple mixtures of a drug(s) in an ointment base. A cream is a semi-solid emulsion. Oleaginous (oil based) bases generally release substances slowly and unpredictably. Water miscible or aqueous bases tend to release drugs more rapidly.

KEY CONCEPTS

Test your knowledge by covering the information in the right hand column.

emulsion	An unstable system consisting of at least two immiscible (unmixable) liquids, one that is dispersed as small droplets throughout the other, and a stabilizing agent.
oil-in-water (o/w)	An emulsion of oils, petroleum hydrocarbons, and/or waxes with water, where the aqueous phase is generally in excess of 45% of the total weight of the emulsion.
water-in-oil (w/o)	When water or aqueous solutions are dispersed in an oleaginous (oil based) medium, with the aqueous phase constituting less than 45% of the total weight.
emulsifiers	Emulsifiers provide a protective barrier around the dispersed droplets that stabilize the emulsion. Commonly used emulsifiers include: tragacanth, sodium lauryl sulfate, sodium dioctyl sulfosuccinate, and polymers known as the Spans and Tweens.
suppository bases	There are three classes that are based on their composition and physical properties: oleaginous bases, water soluble or miscible bases, and hydrophilic bases.
polyethylene glycols (PEGs)	Popular water soluble bases that are chemically stable, non-irritating, miscible with water and mucous secretions, and can be formulated by molding or compression in a wide range of hardnesses and melting points.
fusion molding	A method in which the drug is dispersed or dissolved in a melted suppository base. The fusion method can be used with all types of suppositories and must be used with most of them.
compression molding	A method of preparing suppositories by mixing the suppository base and the drug ingredients and forcing the mixture into a special compression mold.
capsules	When filling, the smallest capsule capable of containing the final volume is used since patients often have difficulty swallowing large capsules.

USING A BALANCE

Class A Balance

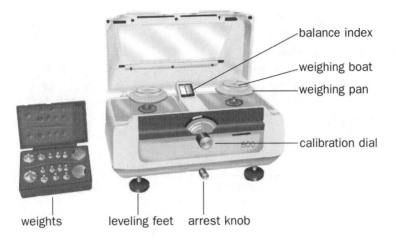

BASIC GUIDELINES FOR USING BALANCES

There are some general rules about using a balance that help to maintain the balance in top condition.

✔ Always cover both pans with weighing papers or use weighing boats. These protect the pans from abrasions, eliminate the need for repeated washing, and reduce loss of drug to porous surfaces.

✔ A clean paper or boat should be used for each new ingredient to prevent contamination of components.

✔ The balance must be readjusted after a new weighing paper or boat has been placed on each pan. Weighing papers taken from the same box can vary in weight by as much as 65 mg. If the new zero point is not established, an error of as much as 65 mg can be made. On 200 mg of material, this is more than 30%. Weighing boats also vary in weight.

✔ Always arrest the balance before adding or removing weight from either pan. Although the balance is noted for its durability, repeated jarring of the balance will ultimately damage the working mechanism of the balance and reduce its accuracy.

✔ Always clean the balance, close the lid, and arrest the pans before storing the balance between uses.

✔ Always use the balance on a level surface and in a draft-free area.

MEASURING

MENISCUS

When reading a volume of a liquid against a graduation mark, hold the graduate so the meniscus is at eye level and read the mark at the bottom of the meniscus. Viewing the level from above will create the incorrect impression that there is more volume in the graduate. If the container is very narrow, the meniscus can be quite large.

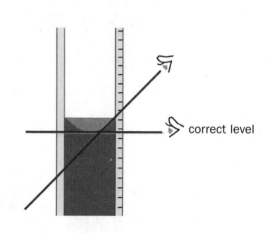

correct level

SYRINGE

When reading a volume of a liquid in a syringe, read to the edge of the stopper.

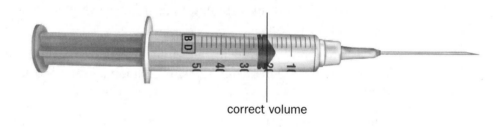

correct volume

CAPSULE SIZES

The relative sizes and fill capacities of capsules are:

Size	Volume (ml)
000	1.37
00	0.95
0	0.68
1	0.5
2	0.37
3	0.3
4	0.2
5	0.13

the punch method
of filling capsules

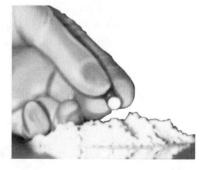

TRUE/FALSE

Indicate whether the statement is true or false in the blank. Answers are at the end of the book.

_____ 1. Compounding must always be done upon receipt of a prescription, never in advance.

_____ 2. Quantities smaller than 120 mg should be weighed on an electronic or analytical balance.

_____ 3. Cylindrical graduates are more accurate than conical ones.

_____ 4. Prescription bottles can be used as volumetric glassware.

_____ 5. Disposable syringes are generally used for measuring small volumes.

_____ 6. When aqueous and non aqueous solutions are mixed, the volume is always equal to the sum of the two volumes.

_____ 7. Levigation is the fine grinding of a powder.

_____ 8. Syrup USP is a supersaturated solution.

_____ 9. In elixirs, alcohol is the solvent for the drug.

_____ 10. With ointments, water miscible bases tend to release drugs more rapidly than oleaginous bases.

_____ 11. An emulsion containing 48% water would be a water-in-oil emulsion.

_____ 12. PEGs of different molecular weight are generally mixed to form a suppository base.

EXPLAIN WHY

Explain why these statements are true or important. Check your answers in the text. Discuss any questions you may have with your Instructor.

1. Why is the stability of a compound important?

2. Why is accuracy in each step of compounding important?

3. Why is the smallest device that will accommodate a volume used to measure it?

4. Why are class A balances not used for very small amounts?

5. Why is geometric dilution used when mixing unequal amounts of powders?

IN THE WORKPLACE

Sample Formulation Record

Formulation Record

Name: _____
Strength: _____
Dosage Form: _____
Route of Administration: _____

Date of Last Review or Revision: _____
Person Completing Last Review or Revision: _____

Formula: [*The formula and all of the information about the individual ingredients are described.*]

Ingredient	Quantity	Physical Description	Solubility	Therapeutic Activity

Example Calculations: [*Examples of calculations that must be made each time the formula is compounded are shown.*]

Equipment Required:

Method of Preparation:

1. [*The method is a step-by-step sequence in the correct order of mixing.*]

2. [*The description of should be clear and detailed so all personnel can complete the step in exactly the same manner.*]

3. [*The description can also consist of graphs, tables, charts, etc.*]

Description of Finished Product:

Formulation Record - Page 2

Name: _____

Strength: _____

Dosage Form: _____

Route of Administration: _____

Quality Control Procedures: [*Details of all quality assurance tests to be performed on final product.*]

Packaging Container:

Storage Requirements:

Beyond-Use Date Assignment: [*Criteria used to assign a beyond-use date.*]

Label Information: [*Auxiliary labels to include.*]

Source of Recipe:

Literature Information: [*Copies of relevant references or primary literature.*]

Sample Compounding Record

Compounding Record

Name: _____

Strength: _____

Dosage Form: _____

Route of Administration: _____

Quantity Prepared: _____

Date of Preparation: _____

Person Preparing Formulation: _____

Person Checking Formulation: _____

Formula: [*This information is completed at the time of compounding.*]

Ingredient	Manufacturer and Lot Number	Purity Grade	Description	Quantity Required	Actual Quantity Used

Calculations: [Calculations performed at the time of compounding.]

Equipment Operation: [*Equipment performance notes or alternate equipment used.*]

Method of Preparation: [*Description of any deviation from the Formulation Record method of preparation.*]

Description of Finished Product:

Quality Control Procedures: [*Details of quality assurance test results and data.*]

Beyond-Use Date Assignment: [*Assigned beyond-use date and reasons for difference from Formulation Record if applicable.*]

IN THE WORKPLACE

Sample Standard Operating Procedure Form.

Standard Operating Procedure

Subject:	Policies and Procedures		
	Effective Date:	Revision Date	Revision No.
	Approved by:	Reviewed by:	
[*What the SOP is concerning*]	[*Additional Items*]	[*Additional Items*]	[*Additional Items*]

Purpose of the SOP: [*Describe the purpose and the desired outcome of the SOP.*]

Procedure:

1.   [*The procedure is a step-by-step sequence in the order of tasks to perform.*]

2.   [*The description of should be clear and detailed so all personnel can complete the step in exactly the same manner*].

3.   [*The description can also consist of graphs, tables, charts, etc.*]

Documentation:

   [*Executing the SOP may generate data or information that needs to be documented. This information may be best reported on a form and maintained in a separate notebook or binder. The form should refer to the execution of the SOP by including the name of the procedure, date it was executed, personnel name conducting the procedure, and then the relevant data or information.*]

FILL IN THE KEY TERM

Answers are at the end of the book.

anticipatory com- pounding	pounding	meniscus	sonication
arrest knob	flocculating agent	miscible	stability
calibrate	formulation record	mucilage	syrup
compression molding	fusion molding	oil-in-water	thickening agent
emulsifier	geometric dilution	primary emulsion	trituration
emulsion	hydrophilic emulsifier	punch method	volumetric
	immiscible	sensitivity require- ment	water-in-oil
	levigation		
extemporaneous com-	lipophilic emulsifier	solvents	

1. _____ : The on-demand preparation of a drug product according to a physician's prescription, formula, or recipe.

2. _____ : The chemical and physical integrity of the dosage unit, and when appropriate, its ability to withstand microbiological contamination.

3. _____ : Compounding in advance of expected need.

4. _____ : To set, mark, or check the graduations of a measuring device.

5. _____ : Measures volume.

6. _____ : The knob on a balance that prevents any movement of the balance.

7. _____ : The curved surface of a column of liquid.

8. _____ : The fine grinding of a powder.

9. _____ : Triturating a powdered drug with a solvent in which it is insoluble to reduce its particle size.

10. _____ : A technique for mixing two powders of unequal size.

11. _____ : Exposure to high frequency sound waves.

12. _____ : Water is the most common, but ethanol, glycerin, propylene glycol, or a variety of syrups are used.

13. _____ : Formulas and procedures of what should happen when a formulation is compounded.

14. _____ : A record of what actually happened when the formulation was compounded.

15. _____ : A concentrated or nearly saturated solution of sucrose in water.

16. _____ : The amount of weight that will move the balance pointer one division mark.

17. _____ : Electrolytes used in the preparation of suspensions.

18. _____ : An agent used in the preparation of suspensions to increase the viscosity of the liquid.

19. _____ : Capable of being mixed together.

20. _____ : Cannot be mixed.

21. _____ : A stabilizing agent in emulsions.

22. _____ : An unstable system consisting of at least two immiscible liquids.

23. _____ : An emulsion in which water is dispersed through an oil base.

24. _____ : An emulsion in which oil is dispersed through a water base.

25. _____ : A stabilizing agent for water based dispersion mediums.

26. _____ : A stabilizing agent for oil based dispersion mediums.

27. _____ : The initial emulsion formed in a preparation to which ingredients are added to create the final volume.

28. _____ : A wet, slimy preparation formed as an initial step in a wet emulsion preparation method.

29. _____ : A method of making suppositories in which the ingredients are compressed in a mold.

30. _____ : A suppository preparation method in which the active ingredients are dispersed in a melted suppository base.

31. _____ : A method for filling capsules by repeatedly pushing or "punching" the capsule into an amount of drug powder.

STUDY NOTES

Use this area to write important points you'd like to remember.

CHOOSE THE BEST ANSWER

Answers are at the end of the book.

1. _____ are used to transfer solid ingredients in compounding
   a. Spatulas
   b. Erlenmeyer flasks
   c. Droppers
   d. Beakers

2. _____ mortars and pestles are preferred for mixing liquid compounds.
   a. Wedgewood
   b. Latex
   c. Glass
   d. Porcelain

3. The minimum weighable quantity for a class A balance is
   a. 120 mg.
   b. 500 ml.
   c. 120 ml.
   d. 500 mg.

4. Metric weights used for weighing ingredients using a class A balance should be handled with
   a. water.
   b. fingers.
   c. forceps.
   d. oil.

5. Quantities less than 120 mg
   a. may be measured using a class A balance.
   b. may be measured using electronic or analytical balances.
   c. may be measured using a class C balance.
   d. may be measured using a class B balance.

6. _____ is the term for triturating a powdered drug with a solvent in which it is insoluble to reduce its particle size.
   a. Suspension
   b. Trituration
   c. Emulsion
   d. Levigation

7. Mixing powders using a spatula is called
   a. extemporaneous compounding.
   b. spatulation.
   c. emulsification.
   d. levigation.

8. A solution that contains the maximum amount of drug it can contain at room temperature is
   a. supersaturated.
   b. saturated.
   c. unsaturated.
   d. eutectic.

9. Syrup USP contains
   a. sucrose in water.
   b. alcohol in water.
   c. oleaginous in water.
   d. PEG in water.

10. _____ are electrolytes used in the preparation of suspensions.
    a. Flocculating agents
    b. Suspending agents
    c. Complex carbohydrates
    d. Simple sugars

11. A two-phase system consisting of a finely divided solid dispersed in a liquid is a/an
    a. suspension.
    b. emulsion.
    c. solution.
    d. trituration.

12. _____ are thickening agents used in the preparation of suspensions.
    a. Electrolytes
    b. Preservatives
    c. Flocculating agents
    d. Suspending agents

13. Cocoa butter is
    a. a water soluble base used for suppositories.
    b. a hydrophilic base used for suppositories.
    c. a water miscible base used for suppositories.
    d. an oleaginous base used for suppositories.

14. The "punch" method is used to prepare
    a. tablets.
    b. capsules.
    c. emulsions.
    d. suppositories.

15. Polyethylene glycol (PEG) polymers are used to make _____ suppositories.
    a. cocoa butter
    b. water soluble or miscible
    c. oleaginous
    d. hydrophilic

16. _____ are mixtures of oleaginous and water miscible bases for making suppositories.
    a. Hydrophobic bases
    b. Hydrophonic
    c. Hydrophilic bases
    d. Hydrotonic bases

STUDY NOTES

Use this area to write important points you'd like to remember.

— 10 —

BASIC BIOPHARMACEUTICS

KEY CONCEPTS

Test your knowledge by covering the information in the right hand column.

objective of drug therapy	To deliver the right drug, in the right concentration, to the right site of action at the right time to produce the desired effect.
receptors	When a drug produces an effect, it is interacting on a molecular level with cell material that is called a receptor. Receptor activation is responsible for most of the pharmacological responses in the body.
site of action	Only those drugs able to bind chemically to the receptors in a particular site of action can produce effects in that site. This is why specific cells only respond to certain drugs.
agonists	Drugs that activate receptors and produce a response that may either accelerate or slow normal cell processes.
antagonists	Drugs that bind to receptors but do not activate them. They prevent other drugs or substances from interacting with receptors.
dose-response curve	Specific doses of a drug is given to various subjects and the effect or response is measured in terms of dose and effect.
blood concentrations	The primary way to monitor a drug's concentration in the body and its related effect is to determine its blood concentrations.
minimum effective concentration (MEC)	When there is enough drug at the site of action to produce a response.
minimum toxic concentration (MTC)	An upper blood concentration limit beyond which there are undesired or toxic effects.

therapeutic window	The range between the minimum effective concentration and the minimum toxic concentration is called the therapeutic window. When concentrations are in this range, most patients receive the maximum benefit from their drug therapy with a minimum of risk.
ADME	Blood concentrations are the result of four simultaneously acting processes: absorption, distribution, metabolism, and excretion.
disposition	Another term for ADME.
elimination	Metabolism and excretion combined.
passive diffusion	Besides the four ADME processes, a critical factor of drug concentration and effect is how drugs move through biological membranes. Most drugs penetrate biological membranes by passive diffusion.
hydrophobic drugs	Lipid (fat) soluble drugs that penetrate the lipoidal (fat-like) cell membrane better than hydrophilic drugs.
hydrophilic drugs	Drugs that are attracted to water.
aqueous pores	Openings in cell membranes that allow entry of water and water soluble drugs.
absorption	The transfer of drug into the blood from an administered drug product is called absorption.
gastric emptying	Most drugs are given orally and absorbed into the blood from the small intestine. One of the primary factors affecting oral drug absorption is the gastric emptying time.
distribution	The movement of a drug within the body once the drug has reached the blood.
selective action	Drug action that is selective to certain tissues or organs, due both to the specific nature of receptor action as well as to various factors that can affect distribution.
protein binding	Many drugs bind to proteins in blood plasma to form a complex that is too large to penetrate cell openings. So the drug remains inactive.
metabolism	The body's process of transforming drugs. The primary site of drug metabolism in the body is the liver. Enzymes produced by the liver interact with drugs and transform them into metabolites.

enzyme	A complex protein that causes chemical reactions in other substances
metabolite	The transformed drug.
enzyme induction	The increase in enzyme activity that results in greater metabolism of drugs.
enzyme inhibition	The decrease in enzyme activity that results in reduced metabolism of drugs.
first-pass metabolism	When a drug is substantially degraded or destroyed by the liver's enzymes before it reaches the circulatory system, an important factor with orally administered drugs.
enterohepatic cycling	The transfer of drugs and their metabolites from the liver to the bile in the gall bladder and then into the intestine.
excretion	The process of excreting drugs and metabolites, primarily performed by the kidney through the urine.
glomerular filtration	The blood filtering process of the kidneys. As plasma water moves through the nephron, waste substances (including drugs and metabolites) are secreted into the fluid, with urine as the end result.
bioavailability	The amount of a drug that is available to the site of action and the rate at which it is available is called the bioavailability of the drug.
bioequivalents	Bioequivalent drug products are pharmaceutical equivalents or alternatives which have essentially the same rate and extent of absorption when administered at the same dose of the active ingredient under similar conditions.
pharmaceutical equivalents	Pharmaceutical equivalents are drug products that contain identical amounts of the same active ingredients in the same dosage form, but may contain different inactive ingredients.
pharmaceutical alternatives	Pharmaceutical alternatives are drug products that contain the identical active ingredients, but not necessarily in the same amount or dosage form.
therapeutic equivalent	Pharmaceutical equivalents that produce the same effects in patients.
therapeutic alternative	Drugs that have different active ingredients but produce similar therapeutic effects.

DOSE RESPONSE CURVE

When a series of specific doses is given to a number of people, the results show that some people respond to low doses but others require larger doses for a response to be produced. Some differences are due to the product itself, but most are due to human variability: different people have different characteristics that affect how a drug product behaves in them. A dose-response curve shows that as doses increase, responses increase up to a point where increased dosage no longer results in increased response.

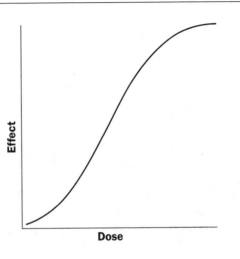

BLOOD CONCENTRATION—TIME PROFILES

Blood concentration begins at zero at the time the drug is administered (before it has been absorbed into the blood). With time, the drug leaves the formulation and enters the blood, causing concentrations to rise. Minimum effective concentration (MEC) is when there is enough drug at the site of action to produce a response. The time this occurs is called the onset of action. With most drugs, when blood concentrations increase, so does the intensity of the effect, since blood concentrations reflect the site of action concentrations that produce the response.

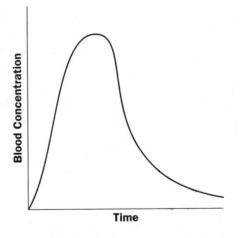

Some drugs have an upper blood concentration limit beyond which there are undesired or toxic effects. This limit is called the minimum toxic concentration (MTC). The range between the minimum effective concentration and the minimum toxic concentration is called the therapeutic window. When concentrations are in this range, most patients receive the maximum benefit from their drug therapy with a minimum of risk.

The last part of the curve shows the blood concentrations declining as absorption is complete. The time between the onset of action and the time when the minimum effective concentration is reached by the declining blood concentrations is called the duration of action. The duration of action is the time the drug should produce the desired effect.

ORAL ABSORPTION

Most drugs are given orally and absorbed into the blood from the small intestine. The small intestine's large surface area makes absorption easier. However, there are many conditions in the stomach that can affect absorption positively or negatively before the drug even reaches the small intestine. One of the primary factors affecting oral drug absorption is the gastric emptying time. This is the time a drug will stay in the stomach before it is emptied into the small intestine. Since stomach acid can degrade many drugs and since most absorption occurs in the intestine, gastric emptying time can significantly affect a drug's action. If a drug remains in the stomach too long, it can be degraded or destroyed, and its effect decreased. Gastric emptying time can be affected by a various conditions, including the amount and type of food in the stomach, the presence of other drugs, the person's body position, and their emotional condition. Some factors increase the gastric emptying time, but most slow it. The pH of the gastrointestinal organs is illustrated at right

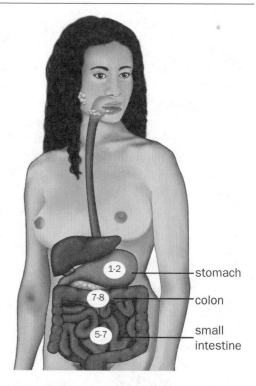

PASSIVE DIFFUSION

Before an effective concentration of a drug can reach its site of action, it must overcome many barriers, most of which are biological membranes, complex structures composed of lipids (fats) and proteins. Most drugs penetrate biological membranes by passive diffusion. This occurs when drugs in the body's fluids move from an area of higher concentration to an area of lower concentration, until the concentrations in each area are in a state of equilibrium. Passive diffusion causes most orally administered drugs to move from the intestine to the blood and from the blood to the site of action.

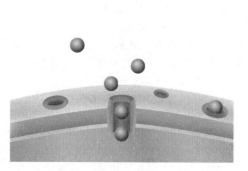

PROTEIN BINDING

Many drugs bind to proteins in blood plasma to form a complex that is too large to penetrate cell openings. So the drug remains inactive. Protein binding can be considered a type of drug storage within the body. Some drugs bind extensively to proteins in fat and muscle, and are gradually released as the blood concentration of the drug falls. These drugs remain in the body a long time, and therefore have a long duration of action.

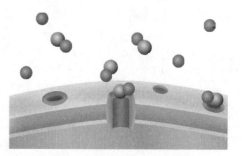

TRUE/FALSE

Indicate whether the statement is true or false in the blank. Answers are at the end of the book.

_____ 1.   Receptors are located on the surfaces of cell membranes and inside cells.

_____ 2.   Agonists may produce a response that slows normal cell process.

_____ 3.   Antagonists bind to cell receptors but do not activate them.

_____ 4.   After all receptors are occupied by a drug, its effect can still be increased by increasing the dose.

_____ 5.   The number or sensitivity of receptors is not affected by prolonged drug use.

_____ 6.   Most patients receive the maximum benefit from drug therapy when the amount of the drug in the blood is between the minimum effective and minimum toxic concentration.

_____ 7.   Passive diffusion is the most common way an orally administered drug is distributed through the body.

_____ 8.   Cell membranes generally absorb hydrophilic drugs more easily than hydrophobic ones.

_____ 9.   Most orally administered drugs are absorbed from the stomach.

_____ 10.   Protein binding can result in the gradual release of a drug into the bloodstream.

_____ 11.   Most drugs and metabolites are excreted by the liver.

EXPLAIN WHY

Explain why these statements are true or important. Check your answers in the text. Discuss any questions you may have with your Instructor.

1.   Why can a drug be developed to have a specific therapeutic effect?

2.   Why can the same drug have different effects in different people?

3.   Why is gastric emptying time important?

4.   Why does the chronic administration of some drugs require increases in dosage to achieve the same effect or decreases to avoid toxicity?

5.   Why is a pharmaceutical equivalent not necessarily therapeutically equivalent?

FILL IN THE KEY TERM

Answers are at the end of the book.

active transport
agonist
antagonist
bioavailability
bioequivalency
biopharmaceutics
complex
disposition
enterohepatic cycling
enzyme

enzyme induction
enzyme inhibition
first pass metabolism
gastric emptying time
glomerular filtration
hydrophilic
hydrophobic
lipoidal
metabolite
minimum effective concentration
nephron

onset of action
passive diffusion
pharmaceutical alternative
pharmaceutical equivalent
protein binding
receptor
selective action
site of action
therapeutic equivalent
therapeutic window

1. _____ : The study of the factors associated with drug products and physiological processes, and the resulting systemic concentrations of the drugs.

2. _____ : The location where an administered drug produces an effect.

3. _____ : The cellular material at the site of action which interacts with the drug.

4. _____ : The characteristic of a drug that makes its action specific to certain receptors and the tissues they affect.

5. _____ : Drugs that activate receptors to accelerate or slow normal cell function.

6. _____ : Drugs that bind with receptors but do not activate them. They block receptor action by preventing other drugs or substances from activating them.

7. _____ : The blood concentration needed of a drug to produce a response.

8. _____ : The time MEC is reached and the response occurs.

9. _____ : A drug's blood concentration range between its minimum effective concentration and minimum toxic concentration.

10. _____ : A term sometimes used to refer to all of the ADME processes together.

11. _____ : The movement of drugs from an area of higher concentration to lower concentration.

12. _____ : The movement of drug molecules across membranes by active means, rather than passive diffusion.

13. _____ : Water repelling; cannot associate with water.

14. _____ : Capable of associating with or absorbing water.

15. _____ : Fat like substance.

16. _____ : The time a drug will stay in the stomach before it is emptied into the small intestine.

17. _____ : Formed when molecules of different chemicals attach to each other, as in protein binding.

18. _____ : The attachment of a drug molecule to a plasma or tissue protein, effectively making the drug inactive, but also keeping it within the body.

19. _____ : The substance resulting from the body's transformation of an administered drug.

20. _____ : A complex protein that causes chemical reactions in other substances.

21. _____ : The increase in enzyme activity that results in greater metabolism of drugs.

22. _____ : The decrease in enzyme activity that results in reduced metabolism of drugs.

23. _____ : The substantial degradation of a drug caused by enzyme metabolism in the liver before the drug reaches the systemic circulation.

24. _____ : The transfer of drugs and their metabolites from the liver to the bile in the gall bladder and then into the intestine.

25. _____ : The functional unit of the kidneys.

26. _____ : The blood filtering process of the kidneys.

27. _____ : The relative amount of an administered dose that reaches the general circulation and the rate at which this occurs.

28. _____ : The comparison of bioavailability between two dosage forms.

29. _____ : Drug products that contain identical amounts of the same active ingredients in the same dosage form.

30. _____ : Drug products that contain the same active ingredients, but not necessarily in the same amount or dosage form.

31. _____ : Pharmaceutical equivalents that produce the same effects in patients.

CHOOSE THE BEST ANSWER

Answers are at the end of the book.

1. _____ are drugs that activate receptors to accelerate or slow normal cellular function.
   a. Channels
   b. Agonists
   c. Antagonists
   d. Protein binding

2. _____ are drugs that bind to receptors but do not activate them.
   a. Channels
   b. Protein binding
   c. Antagonists
   d. Agonists

3. When studying concentration and effect, _____ is the time MEC is reached and the response occurs.
   a. therapeutic window
   b. MTC
   c. onset of action
   d. blood concentration

4. A drug's concentration range between its MEC and MTC is called the
   a. dose response.
   b. therapeutic window.
   c. blood concentration.
   d. onset of action.

5. _____ describes the time following onset of action until the MEC is reached.
   a. Duration of action
   b. Drug concentration
   c. MTC
   d. Onset of action

6. _____ refers to the transfer of drug into the blood from an administered drug product.
   a. Absorption
   b. Excretion
   c. Distribution
   d. Metabolism

7. _____ involves the movement of drugs from an area of lower concentration to an area of higher concentration.
   a. Passive transport
   b. Passive diffusion
   c. Active transport
   d. Absorption

8. One of the primary factors affecting oral drug absorption is
   a. glomerular filtration.
   b. protein binding.
   c. first pass metabolism.
   d. gastric emptying time.

9. The body's process of transforming drugs is called
   a. distribution.
   b. metabolism.
   c. excretion.
   d. absorption.

10. Enterohepatic cycling involves the transfer of drugs and their metabolites from the liver into the
    a. lungs.
    b. peritoneal fluid.
    c. kidneys.
    d. intestine.

11. The _____ filter the blood and remove waste materials from it.
    a. kidneys
    b. liver
    c. gall bladder
    d. small intestine

12. The _____ requires drug manufacturers to perform bioequivalency studies on their products before they are approved for marketing.
    a. DEA
    b. AMA
    c. FDA
    d. United States Pharmacopeia

13. The relative amount of an administered dose that reaches the general circulation and the rate at which this occurs is called
   a. bioavailability.
   b. therapeutic alternative.
   c. bioequivalence.
   d. therapeutic equivalent.

14. Drug products that contain identical amounts of the same active ingredients in the same dosage form are called
   a. alternative drug products.
   b. bioequivalent drug products.
   c. pharmaceutical drug products.
   d. antagonist drug products.

STUDY NOTES

Use this area to write important points you'd like to remember.

– 11 –

FACTORS AFFECTING DRUG ACTIVITY

KEY CONCEPTS

Test your knowledge by covering the information in the right hand column.

human variability	Differences in age, weight, genetics, and gender are among the significant factors that influence the differences in medication responses among people.
age	Drug distribution, metabolism, and excretion are quite different in the neonate and infant than in adults because their organ systems are not fully developed. Children metabolize certain drugs more rapidly than adults. The elderly typically consume more drugs than other age groups. They also experience physiological changes that significantly affect drug action.
pregnancy	A number of physiological changes that occur in women in the latter stages of pregnancy tend to reduce the rate of absorption.
genetics	Genetic differences can cause differences in the types and amounts of proteins produced in the body, which can result in differences in drug action.
pharmacogenetics	A new field of study that defines the hereditary basis of individual differences.
weight	Weight adjustments may be needed for individuals whose weight is more than 50% higher than the average adult weight. Weight adjustments are also made for children, or unusually small, emaciated, or obese adult patients.
allergic reactions	Almost any drug, in almost any dose, can produce an allergic or hypersensitive reaction in a patient. Anaphylactic shock is a potentially fatal hypersensitivity reaction.
common adverse reactions	Anorexia, nausea, vomiting, constipation, and diarrhea are among the most common adverse reactions to drugs.

teratogenicity	The ability of a substance to cause abnormal fetal development when given to pregnant women.
drug-drug interactions	These can result in either increases or decreases in therapeutic effects or adverse effects.
additive effects	Occur when two drugs with similar pharmacological actions are taken, e.g., alcohol and a sedative together produce increased sedation.
synergism or potentiation	Occurs when two drugs with different sites or mechanisms of action produce greater effects when taken together than either does when taken alone, e.g., acetaminophen and codeine together produce increased analgesia.
inhibition	When a drug blocks the activity of metabolic enzymes in the liver.
displacement	Displacement of one drug from protein binding sites by a second drug increases the effects of the displaced drug. Decreased intestinal absorption can occur when orally taken drugs combine to produce nonabsorbable compounds, e.g.. when magnesium hydroxide and oral tetracyline bind.
enzyme induction	Caused when drugs activate metabolizing enzymes in the liver, increasing the metabolism of other drugs affected by the same enzymes.
increased excretion	Some drugs raise urinary pH, lessening renal reabsorption, e.g., sodium bicarbonate raises pH and will cause increased elimination of phenobarbital.
drug-diet interactions	The physical presence of food in the gastrointestinal tract can alter absorption by interacting chemically (e.g., certain medications and tetracycline); improving the water-solubility of some drugs by increasing bile secretion; affecting the performance of the dosage form (e.g., altering the release characteristics of polymer-coated tablets); altering gastric emptying; altering intestinal movement; altering liver blood flow. Some foods contain substances that react with certain drugs, e.g., foods containing tyramine can react with monoamine oxidase (MAO) inhibitors.
disease states	The disposition and effect of some drugs can be influenced by the presence of diseases other than the one for which a drug is used. Hepatic, cardiovascular, renal, and endocrine disease all increase the variability in drug response. For example, decreased blood flow from cardiovascular disorders can delay or cause erratic drug absorption.

FILL IN THE KEY TERM

Answers are at the end of the book.

acute viral hepatitis	displacement	hypothyroidism
additive effects	drug-diet interactions	idiosyncrasy
anaphylactic shock	hepatic disease	inhibition
antidote	hepatotoxity	nephrotoxicity
carcinogenicity	hypersensitivity	synergism
cirrhosis	hyperthyroidism	teratogenicity

1. _____ : An abnormal sensitivity generally resulting in an allergic reaction.

2. _____ : A potentially fatal hypersensitivity reaction producing severe respiratory distress and cardiovascular collapse.

3. _____ : An unexpected reaction the first time a drug is taken, generally due to genetic causes.

4. _____ : Toxicity of the liver.

5. _____ : The ability of a substance to harm the kidneys.

6. _____ : The ability of a substance to cause cancer.

7. _____ : The ability of a substance to cause abnormal fetal development when given to pregnant women.

8. _____ : The increase in effect when two drugs with similar pharmacological actions are taken.

9. _____ : When two drugs with different sites or mechanisms of action produce greater effects when taken together than when taken alone.

10. _____ : When one drug blocks the activity of metabolic enzymes in the liver.

11. _____ : When one drug is moved from protein binding sites by a second drug, resulting in increased effects of the displaced drug.

12. _____ : A drug that antagonizes the toxic effect of another drug.

13. _____ : When elements of ingested nutrients interact with a drug and this affects the disposition of the drug.

14. _____ : A condition in which thyroid hormone secretions are below normal, often referred to as an underactive thyroid.

15. _____ : A condition in which thyroid hormone secretions are above normal, often referred to as an overactive thyroid.

16. _____ : Liver disease.

17. _____ : A chronic and potentially fatal liver disease causing loss of function and resistance to blood flow through the liver.

18. _____ : A virally caused systemic infection that causes inflammation of the liver.

TRUE/FALSE

Indicate whether the statement is true or false in the blank. Answers are at the end of the book.

_____ 1. Human variability is not a significant factor in disposition.

_____ 2. Infants are not able to eliminate drugs as efficiently as adults.

_____ 3. Lower cardiac output in the elderly tends to slow the distribution of drugs.

_____ 4. Commonly used drugs such as acetaminophen and aspirin can produce hepatotoxicity.

_____ 5. Ibuprofen can cause nephrotoxicity.

_____ 6. Analgesics and antihistamines are not considered teratogenic.

_____ 7. Some anticancer drugs are considered carcinogenic.

_____ 8. If one drug interferes with the elimination of another, the effects of the other drug will be decreased.

_____ 9. If one drug displaces another from a protein binding site, the effects of the displaced drug increase.

_____ 10. Cigarette smoking can cause enzyme induction.

EXPLAIN WHY

Explain why these statements are true or important. Check your answers in the text. Discuss any questions you may have with your Instructor.

1. Give at least three reasons why drug-drug interactions can increase the effects of drugs.

2. Give at least three reasons why drug-drug interactions can decrease the effects of drugs.

3. Give at least three reasons diet can affect drug activity.

CHOOSE THE BEST ANSWER

Answers are at the end of the book.

1. Adults experience a decrease in many physiological functions between the ages of
   a. 18 to 30 years.
   b. 20 to 40 years.
   c. 30 to 40 years.
   d. 30 to 70 years.

2. Placebo effects can be due to
   a. pregnancy.
   b. psychological factors.
   c. body weight.
   d. gender.

3. The study of the hereditary basis of individual differences is
   a. lineage.
   b. pharmacoancestry.
   c. pharmacogenetics.
   d. genealogy.

4. Hypersensitivity generally happens because a patient develops
   a. anaphylaxis.
   b. anorexia.
   c. antibodies.
   d. hepatotoxicity.

5. Nephrotoxicity is associated with the
   a. central nervous system.
   b. liver.
   c. kidneys.
   d. small intestine.

6. Idiosyncratic reactions occur the _____ time a drug is given to a patient.
   a. fourth
   b. third
   c. second
   d. first

7. Anticoagulants can cause excessive bleeding and this is an example of
   a. hematological effects.
   b. carcinogenicity.
   c. teratogenicity.
   d. nephrotoxicity.

8. The ability of a substance to cause abnormal fetal development when given to pregnant women is called
   a. hematological effects.
   b. idiosyncrasy.
   c. nephrotoxicity.
   d. teratogenicity.

9. _____ occurs when two drugs with similar pharmacological effects produce greater effects when taken together.
   a. Synergism
   b. Additive effects
   c. Interference
   d. Displacement

10. Drugs that increase activity of metabolizing enzymes in the liver cause
    a. glomerular filtration.
    b. enzyme induction.
    c. renal secretion.
    d. enzyme inhibition.

11. MAO inhibitors interact with some foods to result in
    a. severe hypertension or intracranial hemorrhage.
    b. enzyme induction.
    c. displacement.
    d. anticoagulation.

12. A decrease in kidney function has been correlated with a/an _____ in the elimination of many drugs.
    a. increase
    b. decrease

13. Circulatory disorders are generally charac-
terized by _____ blood flow to
one or more organs.
a. increased
b. decreased

STUDY NOTES

Use this area to write important points you'd like to remember.

— 12 —

INFORMATION

KEY CONCEPTS

Test your knowledge by covering the information in the right hand column.

primary literature	Information based directly on contemporary research.
secondary literature	Primarily general reference works based upon primary literature sources.
tertiary literature	Condensed and compact information based on primary literature.
abstracting services	Services that summarize information from various primary sources for quick reference.
Material Safety Data Sheets (MSDSs)	OSHA required information for handling hazardous chemicals.
state regulations	Many states have laws or State Board of Pharmacy rules and regulations that require pharmacies to maintain specific professional literature references.
Drug Facts and Comparisons (DFC)	A preferred reference for comprehensive and timely drug information, containing information about prescription and OTC products.
Martindale	"The Extra Pharmacopoeia," the best source of information on drugs in clinical use internationally.
Physician's Desk Reference	An annual publication intended for physicians that provides prescription information on major pharmaceutical products.
American Hospital Formulary Service	The authority for drug information questions. It groups drug monographs by therapeutic use.
USP DI	Provides comprehensive and clinically relevant information on drugs in current use.

Handbook on Injectable Drugs	A collection of monographs on commercially available parenteral drugs that include concentration, stability, dosage and compatibility information.
Merck Index	An encyclopedic source of chemical substance data, contains monographs referenced by trade, code, chemical, investigational and abbreviated drug names.
American Drug Index	An exhaustive list of drug products and contains trade and generic drug names, phonetic pronunciations, indications, manufacturers and schedule information in a dictionary format.
Drug Topics Red Book	The pharmacist's guides to products and prices, providing annual price lists of drug products including manufacturer, package size, strength and wholesale and retail prices.
"Orange Book"	The common name for the FDA's Approved Drug Products publication.
Internet	A "supernetwork" of many networks from around the world all connected to each other by telephone lines, and all using a common "language."
search engine	Internet software that searches the Web for specific information you enter.
URLs (uniform resource locators)	The specific addresses of Web sites you want to visit.
personal digital assistants (PDAs)	Small hand-held computers that pharmacists can use for drug information.

STUDY NOTES

Use this area to write important points or Web addresses you'd like to remember.

FILL IN THE KEY TERM

Answers are at the end of the book.

abstracting services
American Hospital Formulary
   Service
browser
Drug Facts and Comparisons

Handbook on Injectable
   Drugs
Internet Service Provider (ISP)
Material Safety Data Sheets
modem
primary literature

secondary literature
tertiary literature
URL
USP DI
World Wide Web

1. _____ : Original reports of clinical and other types of research projects and studies.

2. _____ : Condensed works based on primary literature, such as textbooks, monographs, etc.

3. _____ : Services that summarize information from various primary sources for quick reference.

4. _____ : OSHA required information for handling hazardous chemicals.

5. _____ : General reference works based upon primary literature sources.

6. _____ : The authority for drug information questions. It groups drug monographs by therapeutic use.

7. _____ : A preferred reference for comprehensive and timely drug information, containing information about prescription and OTC products.

8. _____ : Provides comprehensive and clinically relevant information on drugs in current use.

9. _____ : A collection of monographs on commercially available parenteral drugs that include concentration, stability, dosage and compatibility information.

10. _____ : A collection of electronic documents at addresses called Web sites.

11. _____ : A piece of hardware that enables a computer to communicate through telephone lines.

12. _____ : A software program that allows users to view Web sites on the World Wide Web.

13. _____ : A company that provides access to the Internet.

14. _____ : A web address.

TRUE/FALSE

Indicate whether the statement is true or false in the blank. Answers are at the end of the book.

_____ 1. Primary literature is the largest but least current source of information.

_____ 2. MSDS's provide information on the proper protective measures for exposure to hazardous chemicals.

_____ 3. Drug Facts and Comparisons provides information on prescription and OTC drug products, divided into therapeutic groups.

_____ 4. AHSF is a collection of monographs on parenteral drugs.

_____ 5. The PDR is revised once every two years.

_____ 6. The "Orange Book" is included in Volume III of the USP DI: Approved Drug Products and Legal Requirements.

_____ 7. MEDLINE is an annual publication of international medical literature.

_____ 8. The Handbook of Nonprescription Drugs is a comprehensive source of information on OTC products.

_____ 9. A modem is software that allows you to view web sites.

_____ 10. AltaVista is an Internet search engine.

_____ 11. Certified technicians (CPhTs) must obtain 20 hours of continuing education credits every two years to maintain certification.

EXPLAIN WHY

Explain why these statements are true or important. Check your answers in the text. Discuss any questions you may have with your Instructor.

1. Why is primary literature important?

2. Why is continuing education important?

3. Why should technicians be familiar with pharmaceutical information sources?

4. Why should you know how to use an Internet search engine?

CHOOSE THE BEST ANSWER

Answers are at the end of the book.

1. _____ literature contains condensed works based on primary literature, such as textbooks, monographs, etc.
   a. Orange
   b. Secondary
   c. Tertiary
   d. Abstract

2. OSHA requires pharmacies to have _____ for each hazardous chemical on hand.
   a. manufacturer sheets for documentation of safety
   b. Material Safety Data Sheets (MSDSs)
   c. mixture safety documentation sheets
   d. manufacturer's safety documentation sheets

3. _____ contains the USP and NF drug standards and dispensing requirements.
   a. USP DI Volume I
   b. USP DI Volume III
   c. Red Book
   d. Orange Book

4. _____ is the best source of information for drugs used in other countries.
   a. Physicians' Desk Reference
   b. Merck Index
   c. Drug Facts and Comparisons
   d. Martindale: The Extra Pharmacopeia

5. _____ is a collection of monographs on commercially available parenteral drugs.
   a. Merck Index
   b. Orange Book
   c. Handbook of Injectable Drugs
   d. American Drug Index

6. _____ is included in the USP DI Volume III and contains the FDA's approved drug products
   a. The Orange Book
   b. The Red Book
   c. American Drug Index
   d. The Blue Book

7. The Journal of Pharmacy Technology is an example of a
   a. pink sheet.
   b. trade journal.
   c. professional practice journal.
   d. newsletter.

8. The name of the principal pharmacology text is
   a. Goodman and Gilman's
   b. American Drug Index.
   c. Micromedex.
   d. Remington's.

9. A web address is also known as a
   a. url.
   b. dsl.
   c. browser.
   d. isp.

10. The Model Curriculum for Pharmacy Technician Training is published by
   a. APhA.
   b. PTEC..
   c. ASHP
   d. PTCB.

11. CPhT Connection is a newsletter of
   a. PTCB.
   b. PTEC.
   c. ASHP.
   d. APhA.

12. A _____ can be used to search the web for information specified by the user.
   a. modem
   b. browser
   c. search engine
   d. url

13. The Physicians' Desk Reference is published every
   a. month.
   b. 6 months.
   c. year.
   d. two years.

14. _____ is the textbook that would be the best source for information about and OTC product
   a. Orange Book
   b. Red Book
   c. Martindale's
   d. Handbook of Nonprescription Drugs

STUDY NOTES

Use this area to write important points or Web addresses you'd like to remember.

— 13 —

INVENTORY MANAGEMENT

KEY CONCEPTS

Test your knowledge by covering the information in the right hand column.

inventory goals	Good inventory management ensures that drugs which are likely to be needed are both on hand and usable—that is, not expired, damaged, contaminated, or otherwise unfit for use.
open formulary	One that allows purchase of any medication that is prescribed.
closed formulary	A limited list of approved medications.
wholesalers	More than three-quarters of pharmaceutical manufacturers' sales are directly to drug wholesalers, who in turn resell their inventory to hospitals, pharmacies, and other pharmaceutical dispensers. They are government-licensed and regulated.
Schedule II substances	Must be stocked separately in a secure place and require a special order form for reordering. Their stock must be continually monitored and documented.
perpetual inventory	A system that maintains a continuous record of every item in inventory so that it always shows the stock on hand.
spoilage	Inappropriate storage conditions or expired products automatically determine that a product is spoiled since in either case the chemical compounds in the drug product may have degraded.
turnover	The rate at which inventory is used.
point of sale (POS) system	A system in which the item is deducted from inventory as it is sold or dispensed.
drug reorder points	Maximum and minimum inventory levels for each drug.
hard copy	Important reports (especially purchase orders) should be regularly printed out and filed as hard copy both for convenience and as a backup record-keeping system.

computer maintenance

Factors that can damage computer systems are temperature, dust, moisture, movement, vibrations, and power surges.

data back-up

Pharmacy computer files must be regularly backed-up or copied to an appropriate storage media.

order entry device

In a computerized inventory system, a hand-held device to generate orders.

online ordering

In an online ordering system, if an order can be filled as ordered, a message from the supplier will automatically confirm the order to the ordering system. The system automatically assigns to each order a purchase order number for identification.

Material Safety Data Sheets

Instructions for hazardous substances such as chemotherapeutic agents that indicate when special handling and shipping is required.

controlled substance shipping

These substances are shipped separately and checked in by a pharmacist. A special order form must be used for Schedule II substances.

stock bottles

The bulk containers in which most medications are received from the supplier.

storage

Drugs must be stored according to manufacturer's specifications. Most drugs are kept in a fairly constant room temperature of 59°-86°F. The temperature of refrigeration should generally be 36°-46°.

freshness

Medications should be organized in a way that will dispense the oldest items first.

dispensing units

In hospitals and other settings, medications are stocked in dispensing units throughout the facility that may be called supply stations or med-stations.

STUDY NOTES

Use this area to write important points you'd like to remember.

FILL IN THE KEY TERM

Answers are at the end of the book.

closed formulary	order entry device	Schedule II substances
database	perpetual inventory	stock bottles
dispensing units	point of sale system	turnover
open formulary	purchase order number	unit-dose
	reorder points	

1. _____ : One that allows purchase of any medication that is prescribed.

2. _____ : A limited list of approved medications.

3. _____ : The rate at which inventory is used, generally expressed in number of days.

4. _____ : Must be stocked separately in a secure place and require a special order form for reordering. Their stock must be continually monitored and documented.

5. _____ : A system that maintains a continuous record of every item in inventory so that it always shows the stock on hand.

6. _____ : An inventory system in which the item is deducted from inventory as it is sold or dispensed.

7. _____ : Minimum and maximum stock levels which determine when a reorder is placed and for how much.

8. _____ : In a computerized inventory system, a hand-held device to generate orders.

9. _____ : A collection of information structured so that specific information within it can easily be retrieved and used.

10. _____ : A number assigned to each order for products that will allow it to tracked and checked throughout the order process.

11. _____ : The bulk containers in which most medications are received from the supplier.

12. _____ : A package containing a single dose of a medication.

13. _____ : In hospitals and other settings, medications are stocked in units throughout the facility that may also be called supply stations or med-stations.

TRUE/FALSE

Indicate whether the statement is true or false in the blank. Answers are at the end of the book.

_____ 1.   The majority of pharmaceutical manufacturer sales are to wholesalers.

_____ 2.   Drug products can always be sold right up to their date of expiration.

_____ 3.   Reorder points are maximum and minimum inventory levels for a product.

_____ 4.   Computerized ordering systems do not allow manual editing.

_____ 5.   Computers can be adversely affected by dust.

_____ 6.   With computers keeping records, printed copies are not needed.

_____ 7.   Certain hazardous substances may not be shipped by air.

_____ 8.   Schedule II substances may be stored with non-controlled substances.

_____ 9.   Most drug products should be stored at 50°-59°.

_____ 10.   Hospitals frequently use drug dispensing units located at points of use throughout the hospital.

EXPLAIN WHY

Explain why these statements are true or important. Check your answers in the text. Discuss any questions you may have with your Instructor.

1.   Why are wholesalers used?

2.   Why is knowing the turnover rate of a product important?

3.   Why are reorder points used?

4.   Why is it important to make hard copy of computerized reports?

5.   Why is it important to back up computer files?

CHOOSE THE BEST ANSWER

Answers are at the end of the book.

1. The list of medications that are approved for use in a health-care system is called a(an)
   a. turnover.
   b. formulary.
   c. therapeutic equivalent.
   d. wholesaler.

2. Medications that are chemically different but have similar actions and effects are
   a. generic equivalents.
   b. always less expensive.
   c. always more expensive.
   d. therapeutically equivalent.

3. _____ is an expression for the rate at which inventory is used and is generally expressed in number of days.
   a. Reciprocal
   b. Turnover
   c. POS
   d. Availability

4. Portable hand held devices that are widely used to enter ordering data are called
   a. POS machines.
   b. stock machines.
   c. order entry devices.
   d. TI636.

5. Temperature, dust, moisture, movement, vibrations, and power surges _____ computers.
   a. can damage
   b. have no effect on
   c. can enhance
   d. have little effect on

6. Material Safety Data Sheets (MSDS) are required by _____ for hazardous substances and provide hazard, handling, clean-up and first aid information.
   a. OSHA
   b. State Board of Pharmacy
   c. FDA
   d. DEA

7. When reconciling an order, controlled substances are shipped separately, and should be check in by a(an)
   a. technician.
   b. pharmacy clerk.
   c. pharmacist.
   d. intern.

8. _____ are provided by suppliers or wholesalers to return over-shipments, damaged products, or expired products.
   a. Order reports
   b. POS
   c. Return goods forms
   d. Invoices

9. _____ is the term for organizing drugs alphabetically by their generic names.
   a. Unit-Dose
   b. Manufacturer
   c. Point of use
   d. Alpha-generically

10. Stock that is expired should be
    a. left on the regular shelf until two years from the expiration date.
    b. separated from regular stock and clearly marked until it can be returned or destroyed.
    c. left on the regular shelf until one year from the expiration date.
    d. left on the regular shelf until replacement stock arrives.

Study Notes

Use this area to write important points you'd like to remember.

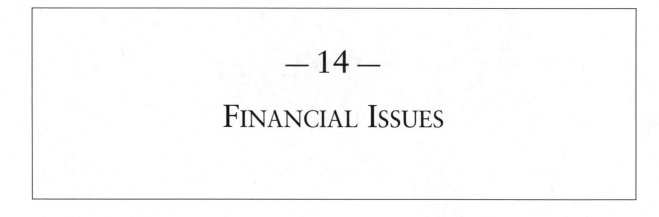

KEY CONCEPTS

Test your knowledge by covering the information in the right hand column.

third party programs

Another party besides the patient or the pharmacy that pays for some or all of the cost of medication: essentially, an insurer.

pharmacy benefit manager (PBM)

A company that administers drug benefit programs for insurance companies, HMOs, and self-insured employers.

co-insurance

Essentially an agreement between the insurer and the insured to share costs.

co-pay

The portion of the cost of prescriptions that patients with third party insurance must pay.

deductible

A set amount that must be paid by the patient for each benefit period before the insurer will cover additional expenses.

maximum allowable cost (MAC)

The amount paid by the insurer is not equal to the retail price normally charged, but is determined by a formula described in a contract between the insurer and the pharmacy. There is a maximum allowable cost (MAC) per tablet or other dispensing unit that an insurer or PBM will pay for a given product.

usual and customary (U&C)

The MAC is often determined by survey of the usual and customary (U&C) prices for a prescription within a given geographic area. This is also referred to as the UCR (usual, customary, and reasonable) price for the prescription.

prescription drug benefit cards

Cards that contain necessary billing information for pharmacies, including the patient's identification number, group number, and co-pay amount.

HMO (health maintenance organization)

Health care networks that usually do not cover expenses incurred outside the network and often require generic substitution.

POS (point of service)	Health care network where the patient's primary care physician must be a member and costs outside the network may be partially reimbursed.
PPO (preferred provider organization)	Health care network that reimburses expenses outside the network at a lower rate than inside the network and usually requires generic substitution.
workers' compensation	Compensation for employees accidentally injured on-the-job.
Medicare	National health insurance for people over the age of 65, disabled people under the age of 65, and people with kidney failure.
Medicaid	A federal-state program for the needy.
online adjudication	Most prescription claims are now filed electronically by online claim submission and online adjudication of claims. In online adjudication, the technician uses the computer to determine the exact coverage for each prescription with the appropriate third party.
dispense as written (DAW)	When brand name drugs are dispensed, numbers corresponding to the reason for submitting the claim with brand name drugs are entered in a DAW (dispense as written) indicator field in the prescription system.
patient identification number	The number assigned to the patient by the insurer that is indicated on the drug benefit card. If it does not match the code for the patient in the insurer's computer (with the same sex and other information) a claim may be rejected.
age limitations	Many prescription drug plans have age limitations for children or dependents of the cardholder.
refills	Most third party plans require that most of the medication has been taken before the plan will cover a refill of the same medication.
maintenance medications	Many managed care health programs require mail order pharmacies to fill prescriptions for maintenance medications.
rejected claims	When a claim is rejected, the pharmacy technician can telephone the insurance plan's pharmacy help desk to determine if the patient is eligible for coverage.

FILL IN THE KEY TERM

Answers are at the end of the book.

co-insurance
co-pay
deductible
dual co-pay
CMS1500 form (formerly
    HCFA 1500 form)
HMOs

maximum allowable cost (MAC)
Medicaid
Medicare
online adjudication
patient assistance programs
patient identification number
pharmacy benefits managers

POSs
PPOs
prescription drug benefit cards
U&C or UCR
universal claim form
workers' compensation

1. _____ : Companies that administer drug benefit programs.

2. _____ : The resolution of prescription coverage through the communication of the pharmacy computer with the third party computer.

3. _____ : An agreement for cost-sharing between the insurer and the insured.

4. _____ : The portion of the price of medication that the patient is required to pay.

5. _____ : Co-pays that have two prices: one for generic and one for brand medications.

6. _____ : The maximum price per tablet (or other dispensing unit) an insurer or PBM will pay for a given product.

7. _____ : The maximum amount of payment for a given prescription, determined by the insurer to be a reasonable price.

8. _____ : A network of providers for which costs are covered inside but not outside of the network.

9. _____ : A network of providers where the patient's primary care physician must be a member and costs outside the network may be partially reimbursed.

10. _____ : A network of providers where costs outside the network may be partially reimbursed and the patient's primary care physician need not be a member.

11. _____ : A set amount that must be paid by the patient for each benefit period before the insurer will cover additional expenses.

12. _____ : Cards that contain third party billing information for prescription drug purchases.

13. _____ : The number assigned to the patient by the insurer that is indicated on the drug benefit card.

14. _____ : A federal program providing health care to people with certain disabilities over age 65.

15. _____ : A federal-state program, administered by the states, providing health care for the needy.

16. _____ : The standard form used by health care providers to bill for services.

17. _____ : An employer compensation program for employees accidentally injured on the job.

18. _____ : Manufacturer sponsored prescription drug programs for the needy.

19. _____ : A standard claim form accepted by many insurers.

TRUE/FALSE

Indicate whether the statement is true or false in the blank. Answers are at the end of the book.

_____ 1.   The amount paid by a co-insurer to the pharmacy is equal to the wholesale price of a drug.

_____ 2.   In online adjudication, the claim processing computer determines if the claim is valid and what the co-pay should be, usually in less than a minute.

_____ 3.   A pharmacy benefits manager is a company that administers drug benefits programs.

_____ 4.   A dual co-pay means that the patient will pay a different co-pay for generic and brand drugs.

_____ 5.   It is up to the pharmacist to decide if generic substitution is available.

_____ 6.   HMOs often require that prescriptions for maintenance medications be filled by a mail order pharmacy.

_____ 7.   All Medicaid programs have an open formulary.

_____ 8.   An NABP number identifies the pharmacy.

EXPLAIN WHY

Explain why these statements are true or important. Check your answers in the text. Discuss any questions you may have with your Instructor.

1. If an online claim is rejected, why is it important to review the information that was originally entered before calling?

2. Why is it important to know the benefits of various third party programs?

CHOOSE THE BEST ANSWER

Answers are at the end of the book.

1. The resolution of prescription coverage for a prescription through the communication of the pharmacy computer with the third party computer is called
   a. PBM.
   b. online adjudication.
   c. MAC.
   d. UCR.

2. The Maximum Allowable Cost (MAC) is usually _____ the Usual and Customary (U&C) price.
   a. less than
   b. greater than
   c. equal to

3. A(an) _____ is a set amount that must be paid by the patient before the insurer will cover additional expenses.
   a. co-insurance
   b. co-pay
   c. maximum allowable cost
   d. deductible

4. A(an) _____ is a network of providers where the patient's primary care physician must be a member and costs outside the network may be partially reimbursed.
   a. HMO
   b. POS
   c. PPO
   d. MAC

5. _____ is a program for people over age 65 or with certain disabilities.
   a. Medicaid
   b. ADC
   c. Workers' Compensation
   d. Medicare

6. Federal and state Workers' Compensation laws include coverage for
   a. HMOs.
   b. accidental injury on-the-job and occupational diseases.
   c. PPOs.
   d. POSs.

7. Procedures for billing compounded prescriptions
   a. should always be referred to the pharmacist.
   b. are not available.
   c. do not apply in community pharmacy practice.
   d. are variable, depending on the insurer or PBM.

8. When a technician receives a rejected claim "invalid birth date", this probably means
   a. the patient has Medicaid.
   b. the patient does not have coverage.
   c. the birth date submitted by the pharmacy does not match the birth date in the insurer's computer.
   d. the patient has Medicare.

9. When a technician receives a rejected claim "Refills Not Covered", this probably means
   a. the plan has a closed formulary.
   b. the patient has a mail order pharmacy for maintenance medications.
   c. the prescriber is not in the network.
   d. the claim may be processed in a few days.

10. Disease Management Services are usually billed
   a. using DEA Form 222.
   b. electronically.
   c. on a universal claim form.
   d. using CMS Form 1500.

STUDY NOTES

Use this area to write important points you'd like to remember.

— 15 —

COMMUNITY PHARMACY

KEY CONCEPTS

Test your knowledge by covering the information in the right hand column.

community pharmacy	The pharmacy practice that provides prescription services to the public. In addition to prescription drugs, community pharmacies sell over-the-counter medications as well as other health and beauty products. In the United States, more than half of all prescription drugs are dispensed by community pharmacies. There are about 60,000 community pharmacies.
counseling	The role of the community pharmacist in counseling and educating patients has been steadily increasing. In the United States, the 1990 Omnibus Budget and Reconciliation Act (OBRA) required community pharmacists to offer counseling to Medicaid patients regarding medications. Many states have expanded this requirement to apply to all customers.
regulation	Community pharmacies are most closely regulated at the state level. In addition to the many regulations on prescribers and prescriptions, states regulations include such things as the ratio of pharmacists to technicians, scope of practice, record keeping, equipment, and work areas.
customer service	A major area of importance in the community pharmacy, since technicians constantly interact with patients as customers. It is important to always respond to customers in a positive and courteous way.
interpersonal skills	Skills involving relationships between people. Good interpersonal skills are based on techniques such as looking the other person in the eye, listening carefully , etc.
telephone use	Telephone calls must be answered in a pleasant and courteous manner, following a standard format that should be indicated by the store manager or pharmacist.

refills	When processing a refill prescription, it is necessary to check that there are refills available. In the case of a patient requesting an early refill of a controlled substance, involve the pharmacist right away.
drug interactions	Whenever the prescription system flags drug interactions and allergy conflicts, alert the pharmacist so that he or she can evaluate the significance of the flag.
safety caps	All dispensed prescription vials and bottles must have a safety cap or child resistant cap, unless the patient requests an easy-open or non-child resistant cap.
auxiliary labels	Auxiliary labels identify important usage information, including specific warnings or alerts on: administration, proper storage, possible side effects, and potential food and drug interactions.
final check by pharmacist	As a final step of the prescription preparation process, the final product and all paperwork, including the original prescription, is organized for the pharmacist's final check.
signature log	Customer signatures in a log are required for Medicaid and most third party insurer or HMO prescriptions, along with Schedule V controlled substances, poisons, and certain other prescriptions (depending upon the state).
mark-up	The amount of the retailer's sale price minus their purchase price. It is calculated by multiplying the retailer's purchase price by the mark-up percentage. For example, a 30% mark-up on an item purchased for $2.30 is $0.69 (2.30 x 0.3), so the sale price would be $2.99.
OTC products	Drug products that do not require a prescription, but are not without risks. Therefore, the technician should not recommend them to pharmacy customers.
shelf stickers	Stickers for OTC drugs and other products that can be scanned for inventory identification.
unit price	The price of a single unit of a product, such as for one ounce of a liquid cold remedy.
stock	Managing stock is often a technician responsibility and includes ordering, receiving, storing, and placing products on shelves.
Disease State Management	Consultation services targeted toward improved therapy of a chronic disease that may be billed to a patient's major medical insurance.

IN THE WORKPLACE

Use these tools to practice and check some of your workplace skills.

Pharmacy Technician Skills Checklist
BASIC COMPUTER ENTRY SKILLS

Name: _____

Skill or Procedure	Self-Assessment		Supervisor Review		
	Needs to Improve	Meets or Exceeds	Needs to Improve*	Meets or Exceeds	*Plan of Action
1. Properly interprets medical abbreviations.					
2. Understands dosage forms.					
3. Understands prescription number assignments (controlled, non-controlled).					
4. Properly enters a new patient into computer.					
5. Properly adds a new patient to an existing family file.					
6. Properly uses SIG codes.					
7. Properly adds medication allergy codes.					
8. Properly processes refill prescriptions using computer.					
9. Understands procedures for DUR screens.					
10. Properly enters third party billing (insurance) information.					
11. Properly adds a new doctor file (if doctor is not already in the database).					
12. Chooses correct drug (matches NDC).					
13. Uses appropriate DAW codes.					

Name: _____

Pharmacy Technician Skills Checklist
GENERAL COMPUTER ENTRY SKILLS

Skill or Procedure	Self-Assessment		Supervisor Review		
	Needs to Improve	Meets or Exceeds	Needs to Improve*	Meets or Exceeds	*Plan of Action
1. Properly puts new prescriptions on file (without filling).					
2. Enters and uses alternate third party plans.					
3. Enters compounded prescriptions.					
4. Generates daily reports.					
5. Generates medical expense statements.					
6. Updates inventories.					
7. Updates order quantities.					

FILL IN THE KEY TERM

Answers are at the end of the book.

auxiliary labels   group number   safety caps
bar code   interpersonal skills   signa
confidentiality   OBRA '90   scope of practice
counting tray   patient identification number   shelf stickers
DEA number   refrigeration   unit price

1. _____ : Required community pharmacists to offer counseling to Medicaid patients regarding medications.

2. _____ : Based on techniques such as looking the other person in the eye, listening carefully, etc.

3. _____ : What technicians may and may not do, as mandated by their state.

4. _____ : The requirement to keep patient information private between the patient and the patient's care providers.

5. _____ : Temperature should be between 2°-8° C (36°-46°F).

6. _____ : The number of the patient's insurance policy as indicated on their drug benefit card.

7. _____ : A number that identifies a patient's employer.

8. _____ : Directions for use.

9. _____ : Required for all controlled substance prescriptions and by many third party insurers.

10. _____ : Child resistant caps required of all dispensed prescription vials.

11. _____ : A tray designed for counting pills.

12. _____ : Stickers with product information that can be scanned for inventory identification.

13. _____ : A series of lines that identify a product when scanned.

14. _____ : Labels regarding specific warnings and usage information.

15. _____ : For example, the price for one ounce of a liquid cold remedy.

TRUE/FALSE

Indicate whether the statement is true or false in the blank. Answers are at the end of the book.

_____ 1. More than half of all drugs in the U.S. are sold at community pharmacies.

_____ 2. Many states put limits on the number of technicians assisting the pharmacist at a given time.

_____ 3. It is important to get the prescription number for refills.

_____ 4. The DAW code is only required for controlled substance prescriptions.

_____ 5. It is up to the pharmacist to decide the number of refills.

_____ 6. Safety caps are not used for patients who request an easy open cap.

_____ 7. When the computerized prescription system flags a drug interaction or allergy, the person to tell this to is the patient.

_____ 8. When a technician prepares a prescription, it is always checked by the pharmacist before dispensing to the patient.

_____ 9. Medicaid requires signatures for dispensed prescriptions.

_____ 10. OTC products may be purchased without a prescription because they are without risk.

_____ 11. Expired drugs must either be returned to the wholesaler or destroyed.

EXPLAIN WHY

Explain why these statements are true or important. Check your answers in the text. Discuss any questions you may have with your Instructor.

1. Why is the health of customers a factor in community pharmacy?

2. Why are good interpersonal skills important in community pharmacy?

3. Why is it important to look a patient in the eye and restate what they have said?

4. Why does the pharmacist check technician filled prescriptions before dispensing to patients?

5. Why shouldn't technicians recommend OTC products?

CHOOSE THE BEST ANSWER

Answers are at the end of the book.

1. Community pharmacies within stores like Walmart or KMart, that are part of regional or national mass merchandise chains are
   a. chain pharmacies.
   b. mass merchandiser pharmacies.
   c. independent pharmacies.
   d. food store pharmacies.

2. Customer service is a major area of importance in _____ compared to _____.
   a. community pharmacy, institutional pharmacy
   b. hospital pharmacy, institutional pharmacy
   c. institutional pharmacy, community pharmacy
   d. institutional pharmacy, hospital pharmacy

3. The refrigerator in a community pharmacy must store medications between
   a. 2 and 8 degrees Fahrenheit.
   b. 32 and 40 degrees Celsius.
   c. 2 and 8 degrees Celsius.
   d. 32 and 40 degrees Fahrenheit.

4. Techniques for interacting with customers on the telephone include
   a. listening carefully, making eye contact, repeating what the customer has said, and using positive language to describe what you can do.
   b. using a pleasant and courteous manner, stating the name of the pharmacy and your name, following the standard procedure indicated for your pharmacy, and referring all calls that require a pharmacist's judgment to the pharmacist.

5. If a patient is requesting a refill, the technician should be sure to obtain the
   a. patient's name and prescription number.
   b. correct drug and strength, correct physician's name, directions for use, quantity, number of refills, DAW code, and initials of the dispensing pharmacist.

6. The final check of a new prescription is performed by
   a. the pharmacist.
   b. the prescribing physician.
   c. a certified technician.
   d. the senior technician.

7. OTC product recommendations should be made by
   a. certified technicians.
   b. technicians with seniority.
   c. pharmacists.
   d. technicians with more than two years of experience.

8. When receiving orders for Schedule II controlled substances, they must be checked and signed by the
   a. certified pharmacy technician.
   b. pharmacy technician.
   c. pharmacist.
   d. third party.

9. Disease state management services may be billed directly to the patient or to
   a. universal claim forms.
   b. major medical insurance.
   c. the primary care physician.
   d. the prescribing physician.

10. Teaching a patient how to use a blood glucose meter in a disease state management program is a duty of the
    a. certified pharmacy technician.
    b. third party.
    c. pharmacist.
    d. pharmacy technician.

STUDY NOTES

Use this area to write important points you'd like to remember.

— 16 —

INSTITUTIONAL PHARMACY

KEY CONCEPTS

Test your knowledge by covering the information in the right hand column.

around-the-clock care

Hospitals provide care around the clock. Standard shifts are 7am to 3:30pm; 3:00pm to 11:30pm; and 11:00pm to 7:00am.

patient care units

Patient rooms are divided into groups called nursing units or patient care units, with patients having similar problems often located on the same unit.

nurse's station

The work station for medical personnel on a nursing unit is called the nurse's station. Various items required for care of patients are stored there, including patient medications.

ancillary areas

Areas such as the emergency room that also use medications and are serviced by the pharmacy department.

centralized pharmacy

A system in which all pharmacy activities are conducted from one location within the hospital: the inpatient pharmacy.

decentralized pharmacy

A system in which there are several pharmacy areas (called satellites) located throughout the hospital, each performing a specific function.

investigational drug service

A specialized pharmacy subsection that deals solely with clinical drug trials. These drug studies require a great deal of paperwork and special documentation of all doses of medication taken by patients. Technicians frequently assist the pharmacist with this documentation and in preparing individual patient medication supplies.

pharmacist supervision

Pharmacy technicians in the hospital work under the direct supervision of a pharmacist. Only a pharmacist may verify orders in the computer system and check medications being sent to the nursing floors.

formulary	A list of drugs stocked at the hospital which have been selected based on therapeutic factors as well as cost.
closed-formulary	A closed formulary means that a hospital carries only formulary medications and physicians must order from this list.
non-formulary	Drugs not on the formulary list.
patient drug profiles	Computer generated drug profiles are prepared daily for each patient
patient medication trays	The amount of medications for a 24 hour period are placed in patient trays that are loaded into medication carts.
unit doses	The amount of drug required for one dose, called a unit dose.
unit dose labels	Unit dose labels contain bar codes for identification and control. Items are scanned into the dispensing and inventory system at various stages up to dispensing. This reduces the chances of medication errors and improves documentation and inventory control.
pre-packing	Technicians often "pre-pack" medications that have been supplied in bulk into unit doses. Machines that automate this process are generally used for pre-packing oral solid medications.
medication order form	In the hospital, all drugs ordered for a patient are written on a medication order form and not a prescription blank as in a community pharmacy. Physicians write medication orders for hospital patients, though both nurses and pharmacists may also write orders if they are directly instructed to do so by a doctor. In addition, physician's assistants and nurse practitioners may sometimes write orders, depending upon the institution.
medication administration record	Nurses record and track medication orders on a patient specific form called the medication administration record (MAR).
physician order entry	A computer system that allows the physician to enter the medication order directly into the hospital computer system.
controlled substances	A primary area of concern for inventory control is narcotics, or controlled substances, which require an exact record of the location of every item to the exact tablet or unit.
code carts	Locked carts filled with emergency medications. All patient care areas are required to have code carts.

KEY CONCEPTS

Test your knowledge by covering the information in the right hand column.

IV admixtures	A large portion of the medication used in the hospital is administered intravenously. Pharmacy technicians prepare I.V. admixtures, including small and large volume parenterals, enteral nutrition therapy, and chemotherapy.
policy and procedures manual	A manual containing information about every aspect of the job from dress code to disciplinary actions and step by step directions on how to perform various tasks that will be required of technicians. All departments within the hospital are required by regulating agencies to maintain this.
JCAHO	The Joint Commission on Accreditation of Healthcare Organizations, the accreditation agency for healthcare organizations. Organizations undergo a JCAHO survey every 3 years.
long-term care	Facilities that provide care for people unable to care for themselves because of mental or physical impairment. Because of limited resources, most long-term care facilities will contract out dispensing and clinical pharmacy services.
distributive pharmacist	A long-term care pharmacist responsible for making sure patients receive the correct medicines that were ordered.
consultant pharmacist	A long-term care pharmacist who develops and maintains an individualized pharmaceutical plan for every long-term care resident.
emergency kits	Locked kits containing emergency medications, similar to code carts used in hospitals.
automated dispensing stations	Automated units which dispense medications at the point of use.

unit dose medications

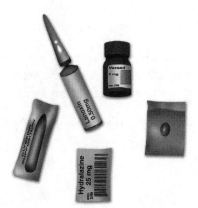

patient trays

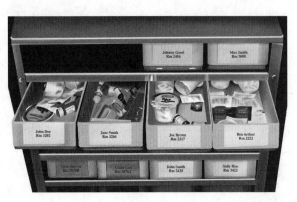

MEDICATION ORDERS

Medication order forms are an all-purpose communication tool used by the various members of the healthcare team. Orders for various procedures, laboratory tests, and x-rays may be written on the form in addition to medication orders. Several medication orders may be written on one medication order form unlike pharmacy prescription blanks seen in the retail setting.

There are several different types of orders that can be written. One is a standard medication order for patients to receive a certain drug at scheduled intervals throughout the day, sometimes called a standing order. Orders for medications that are administered only on an as needed basis are called PRN medication orders. A third type of order is for a medication that is needed right away and these are referred to as STAT orders.

COMMUNITY HOSPITAL
Medication Administration Record

Room/Bed: 675-01
Patient: SMITH, JOHN
Account #: 099999999
Sex: M
Age: 48Y
Doctor: JOHNSON, P.

From 0730 on 02/01/04 to 0700 on 02/02/04

Diagnosis: PNEUMONIA; DEHYDRATION
Height: 5'11" weight: 75KG

Verified By: *Susie Smith, RN*

Allergies: PENICILLIN-->RASH

	0730–1530	1600–2300	2330–0700
0.9% SODIUM CHLORIDE 1 LITER BAG DOSE 125 ML/HR IV ORDER #2	800 JD	1600 SS	2400
MULTIVITAMIN TABLET DOSE: 1 TABLET P.O. QD ORDER #4	* 1000 Given 9AM JD		
CLARITHROMYCIN 500 MG TABLET DOSE: 500MG P.O. Q 12 HRS ORDER #5	1000 JD	2200 SS	
ACETAMINOPHEN 325 MG TABLET DOSE: 650 MG P.O. Q 4-6 H P.R.N. FOR TEMP>38°C ORDER # 17	1200 JD		

Init / Signature
SS / Susie Smith, RN
JD / Jane Doe, RN
____ / _____

Init / Signature
____ / _____
____ / _____
____ / _____

MEDICATION ADMINISTRATION RECORD

On this form every medication ordered for a patient is written down as well as the time it is administered and the person who gave the dose. These forms may be handwritten by the nursing staff or generated by the pharmacy computer system. The MAR is an important document in tracking the care of the patient as it gives a 24 hour picture of a patient's medication use. The accuracy of this document is crucial.

MEDICATION ADMINISTRATION RECORD FORM #M-12

ALLERGIES
PCN → Rash

INJECTION SITE(S)
a. RT DELT e. RT THIGH
b. LT DELT f. LT THIGH
c. RT GLUT g. RT ABD
d. LT GLUT h. ABD

REASON MED NOT GIVEN
1. NPO
2. Off Unit
3. Pt. refused
4. Drug not available
5. Nauseated
6. Other-specify above X

DIAGNOSIS:

R	ORD #	ORDER	DOSE	RT	FREQN	8 9 0 1 2 3 4 5	5 7 8 9 0 1 2 3	0 1 2 3 4 5 6 7
	1378	Clarithromycin (Biaxin)	500 mg tab	PO	q 12°	X JD	X SS	
	1379	Multivitamin	1 tab	PO	qd	X JD		
	1380	5% Dextrose 109% Sod Chloride 1 liter	125 ml/hr	IV	q 8°	X JD	X JD	X
	1402	Acetaminophen (tylenol) PRN for Temp >38°C	650 mg	PO	q 4-6°	X JD		

INITIALS SIGNATURE
SS Susie Smith, RN
JD Jane Doe, RN

INITIALS SIGNATURE

NAME: Smith, John   ACCT #: 099999999
ROOM #: 675-01
MEDICATION SCHEDULE FROM: 2/01/04   THROUGH: 2/02/04

FILL IN THE KEY TERM

Answers are at the end of the book.

automated dispensing system
centralized pharmacy system
clean rooms
code carts
consultant pharmacist
decentralized pharmacy system
distributive pharmacist

inpatient pharmacy
Licensed Practical Nurse,
   L.P.N.
medication administration
   record (MAR)
Nurse Practitioner
outpatient pharmacy

policy and procedure manual
PRN order
Registered Nurse, R.N.
satellites
standing order
STAT order
unit dose

1. _____ : A registered nurse with additional training who can provide basic primary health care. The N.P. can prescribe various medications in most states.

2. _____ : A nurse who provides bedside care, assists physicians in various procedures, and administers medical regimens to patients.

3. _____ : A nurse who is not allowed to perform all functions of an R.N. and may not administer medication to patients.

4. _____ : A package containing the amount of a drug required for one dose.

5. _____ : A standard medication order for patients to receive medication at scheduled intervals.

6. _____ : An order for medication to be administered only on an as needed basis.

7. _____ : An order for medication to be administered immediately.

8. _____ : A form that tracks the medications administered to a patient.

9. _____ : A locked cart of medications designed for emergency use only.

10. _____ : A system in which all pharmacy activities in the hospital are conducted at one location, the inpatient pharmacy.

11. _____ : The hospital pharmacy in a centralized system.

12. _____ : A system in which pharmacy activities occur in multiple locations within a hospital.

13. _____ : A list of drugs stocked at the hospital based on cost and therapeutic factors.

14. _____ : Areas designed for the preparation of sterile products.

15. _____ : A pharmacy attached to a hospital servicing patients who have left the hospital or who are visiting doctors in a hospital outpatient clinic.

16. _____ : Documentation of required policies, procedures, and disciplinary actions in a hospital.

17. _____ : Makes sure long-term care patients receive the correct medications ordered.

18. _____ : Develops and maintains an individual pharmaceutical plan for each long-term care patient.

19. _____ : Automated unit which dispenses medications at the point of use.

TRUE/FALSE

Indicate whether the statement is true or false in the blank. Answers are at the end of the book.

_____ 1. An LPN supervises a Nurse Practitioner in the hospital setting.

_____ 2. Orders for medications that are needed immediately are PRN orders.

_____ 3. Technicians often prepare IV admixtures in hospitals.

_____ 4. Oral medications in hospitals are delivered to patient care areas in carts containing patient specific trays.

_____ 5. A centralized pharmacy system is made up of an inpatient pharmacy and satellite pharmacy areas.

_____ 6. All departments within a hospital are required to maintain a policy and procedure manual.

_____ 7. The consultant pharmacist develops and maintains an individual pharmaceutical plan for each long-term care patient.

EXPLAIN WHY

Explain why these statements are true or important. Check your answers in the text. Discuss any questions you may have with your Instructor.

1. Why can several medication orders be written on a single medication order form?

2. Why is it important for technicians to be familiar with the policy and procedures manual for their department?

CHOOSE THE BEST ANSWER

Answers are at the end of the book.

1. The central area of the hospital responsible for distributing supplies to all areas of the facility is called (the)
   a. centralized pharmacy.
   b. central supply or materials management.
   c. decentralized pharmacy.
   d. satellite pharmacy.

2. A trained individual who assists in the evaluation, treatment, and care of patients with breathing problems or illnesses is a(an)
   a. P.T.
   b. R.T.
   c. P.A.
   d. N.P.

3. A health care provider who is concerned with factors such as a patient's ability to pay for medications is a(an)
   a. Pharm.D.
   b. R.Ph.
   c. N.P.
   d. M.S.W.

4. A nurse who provides basic bedside care under the supervision of an R.N. is a(an)
   a. L.P.N.
   b. R.T.
   c. N.P.
   d. R.D.

5. The person in the medical staff who coordinates care for patients under close supervision of a physician is a(an)
   a. P.A.
   b. P.T.
   c. R.T.
   d. L.P.N.

6. The healthcare worker that provides services to help restore function, improve mobility, relieve pain, and prevent or limit permanent physical disabilities of patients is
   a. Pharm.D.
   b. R.T.
   c. N.P.
   d. P.T.

7. Each individual drawer in a medication cart is filled with
   a. the most commonly used medications for a given floor.
   b. large volume parenteral that do not require patient specific labeling.
   c. controlled substances only.
   d. daily medication for a given patient.

8. Verbal orders must be signed by the nurse or pharmacist who took the verbal order and cosigned by the _____ who approved them.
   a. P.T.
   b. physician
   c. R.T.
   d. M.S.W.

9. Orders for medications that are needed right away are called
   a. PRN orders.
   b. parenteral.
   c. STAT orders.
   d. standing orders.

10. A locked cart of medications designed for emergency use is called a
    a. PCU.
    b. code cart.
    c. satellite.
    d. IP.

11. Rooms designed for the preparation of sterile products are called
    a. satellites.
    b. clean rooms.
    c. CPs.
    d. PCUs.

12. Which of the following agencies is responsible for approving hospitals so they may receive Medicaid reimbursement?
    a. BOP
    b. JCAHO
    c. HCFA
    d. DPH

STUDY NOTES

Use this area to write important points you'd like to remember.

— 17 —

OTHER ENVIRONMENTS

KEY CONCEPTS

Test your knowledge by covering the information in the right hand column.

mail order pharmacy	Delivery of prescriptions by mail (primarily for maintenance therapy). Mail order pharmacies are generally large scale operations that are highly automated. They use assembly line processing in which each step in the prescription fill process is completed or managed by a person who specializes in that step.
maintenance therapy	Therapy for chronic conditions that include depression, gastrointestinal disorders, heart disease, hypertension and diabetes.
regulation	Mail order pharmacies must follow federal and state requirements in processing prescriptions, but are not necessarily licensed in each state to which they send medications.
pharmacist review	Pharmacists review mail order prescriptions before and after filling.
on-line drugstore	A type of mail order pharmacy that uses the internet to advertise and take orders for drugs.
home care	Care in the home, generally supervised by a registered nurse who works with a physician, pharmacist, and others to administer a care plan that involves the patient or another care giver.
home infusion	Infusion administered in the home, the fastest growing area of home health care. The primary therapies provided by home infusion services are: antibiotic therapy, parenteral nutrition, pain management and chemotherapy.
infusion pumps	Pumps that control infusion. There are pumps for specific therapies or multiple therapies, as well as ambulatory pumps that can be worn by patients.
patient education	In home infusion, the patient or their care giver is educated about their therapy: how to self-administer, monitor, report problems, and so on.

admixture preparation   The same rules apply to preparing parenteral admixtures in the home infusion setting as in the hospital.

TRUE/FALSE

Indicate whether the statement is true or false in the blank. Answers are at the end of the book.

_____ 1.   A chronic condition is a serious condition that requires acute care therapy.

_____ 2.   Mail order pharmacies are often used to handle maintenance medications.

_____ 3.   Community pharmacy is growing more rapidly than mail order pharmacy.

_____ 4.   Antibiotic therapy is a common home infusion service used in treating AIDS related and other infections.

_____ 5.   On the home care team, the technician works under the supervision of a home care aide.

_____ 6.   In home infusion, waste from chemotherapy and the treatment of AIDS patients can be safely disposed with the patient's other trash.

_____ 7.   Pain management generally applies to the infusion of narcotics for patients with painful terminal illnesses or other types of severe chronic pain.

_____ 8.   In home infusion, the stability of the admixture is a primary concern.

EXPLAIN WHY

Explain why these statements are true or important. Check your answers in the text. Discuss any questions you may have with your Instructor.

1.   Why is mail order pharmacy growing so rapidly?

2.   Why would maintenance drugs be well suited to mail order delivery?

3.   Why is patient education important in home infusion?

4.   Why is home infusion growing so rapidly?

5.   Why is storage of admixtures an issue in home infusion?

6.   Why is hazardous waste an issue in home infusion?

CHOOSE THE BEST ANSWER

Answers are at the end of the book.

1. In the U.S., a mail order pharmacy can provide services to
   a. only the states where the company has pharmacies.
   b. only the state of the main campus.
   c. only the state of the main campus and adjacent states.
   d. any state in the U.S.

2. A medication that is required on a continuing basis for the treatment of a chronic condition is called
   a. PRN medication.
   b. PO medication.
   c. STAT medication.
   d. maintenance medication.

3. Medication counseling for mail order pharmacies is done by
   a. registered nurses.
   b. certified technicians.
   c. nurses.
   d. pharmacists.

4. For home infusions, the pharmacist consults with the _____ to choose the appropriate pump.
   a. supervising nurse
   b. physician
   c. home care aide
   d. pharmacy technician

5. Home care nursing businesses that provide a range of health care services are
   a. home care agencies.
   b. nursing homes.
   c. CCUs.
   d. hospitals.

6. The type of infusion therapy that usually involves infusion of narcotics for patients with painful terminal illness or severe chronic pain is called
   a. laxative therapy.
   b. maintenance therapy.
   c. pain management therapy.
   d. infection therapy.

7. Regulation of hazardous waste procedures associated with chemotherapy applies to all of the following EXCEPT:
   a. storage.
   b. disposal.
   c. transportation.
   d. pricing.

8. Which member of the home care team is responsible for educating the patient?
   a. R.Ph.
   b. physician
   c. registered nurse
   d. Pharm.D.

9. Which member of the home care team is non-professional staff?
   a. home care aide
   b. pharmacist
   c. pharmacy technician
   d. physician

10. Which of the following activities would NOT be part of the pharmaceutical care plan for home infusion pharmacy?
   a. identification of adverse reactions and interventions
   b. delivery
   c. medication monitoring practices
   d. selection of infusion device

STUDY NOTES

Use this area to write important points you'd like to remember.

— Appendix A —

DRUG CLASSIFICATIONS

CLASSIFICATION OF DRUGS

There are thousands of drugs used in pharmacy. A basic familiarity with these drugs and their uses will enhance your skills as a pharmacy technician.

Drugs may be classified in different ways. One way is *based on their main therapeutic indication or action.* An example of such a group name would be **antibiotic,** which describes drugs that work by destroying pathogenic organisms (microorganisms that cause disease). Another example of a group name would be **analgesic,** which describes drugs that are used in the alleviation of pain. Following is a sample list of such group names:

Analgesics	Hematological Agents
Anesthetics	Hormones & Modifiers
Anti-infectives	Immunobiologic Agents
Antineoplastic Agents	Musculoskeletal Agents
Cardiovascular Agents	Neurologic Agents
Dermatologicals	Ophthalmic Agents
Electrolytes	Psychotropic Agents
Gastrointestinal Agents	Respiratory Agents

Another arrangement of drugs is by *specific classification based on how the drug actually works.* Drugs classified this way generally share these characteristics:

1. similar chemical structure
2. similar mechanism of action
3. similar effects (including side effects)

An example of such a classification is the **cephalosporins,** which is found in the antibiotics group. Drugs in the cephalosporins classification share the above mentioned characteristics with each other but not necessarily with other antibiotics, which may have different characteristics. Another example of such a group would be **xanthine derivatives,** which are found in the bronchodilators group.

Example:

Trade Name	Generic Name	Group	Classification
Keflex	Cephalexin	Antibiotic	Cephalosporin
Theo-Dur	Theophylline	Bronchodilator	Xanthine Derivative

Below is a sample list of such classifications:

Angiotensin Converting Enzyme inhibitors (ACE inhibitors)
α-adrenergic agonists
β-blockers
Calcium channel blockers
Cephalosporins
Corticosteroids
Histamine$_2$ blockers
Loop Diuretics

For the National Pharmacy Technician Certification Exam, you will need to know the main groups of drugs used in the retail and hospital setting. More specific classifications are not emphasized. You will learn most of this information on the job: as you handle these medications over and over again, you'll see which drugs are the most commonly used and which are not.

STUDY NOTES

Use this area to write important points you'd like to remember.

COMMON DRUGS

The following are common drugs listed by classification, generic names, and a limited description of their therapeutic use.

ANALGESICS

Acetylsalicylic Acid (Aspirin)	antipyretic, pain relieving, anti-inflammatory, and anticoagulant.
Methyl Salicylate	topical anti-inflammatory.
Acetaminophen	antipyretic, pain relieving.
Ibuprofen	antipyretic, pain relieving, anti-inflammatory agent.
Nabumetone	non-steroidal anti-inflammatory (NSAID) pain relieving agent.
Naproxen	NSAID, anti-inflammatory, pain relieving.
Oxaprozin	long acting anti-inflammatory, antipyretic, pain relieving agent.
Tramadol Hydrochloride	serotonin reuptake inhibitor for moderate to severe pain.
Hydrocodone Bitartate & Acetaminophen	a narcotic analgesic.
Morphine Sulfate	a narcotic analgesic.
Meperidine Hydrochloride	synthetic opioid analgesic.
Propoxyphene Hydrochloride	mild narcotic analgesic.

ANESTHETICS

Procaine	injection local anesthetic.
Tetracaine	injection local anesthetic.
Bupivacaine	injection local anesthetic.
Dibucaine	injection local anesthetic.
Nitrous Oxide	inhalation general anesthetic.
Halothane	inhalation general anesthetic.
Midazolam	injectable general anesthetic.
Fentanyl Citrate/Droperidol	injectable general anesthetic.

ANTI-INFECTIVES

Ampicillin	penicillin-like antibiotic.
Amoxicillin / Clavulanate	semi-synthetic antibiotic.
Cerufoxime Axetil	cephalosporin antibiotic.
Cefprozil Monohydrate	cephalosporin antibiotic.
Cefaclor	cephalosporin antibiotic.
Cephalexin Hydrochloride	cephalosporin antibiotic.
Levofloxacin	quinolone antibiotic.
Ciprofloxacin	quinolone antibiotic.
Azithromycin	macrolide antibiotic.
Clarithromycin	macrolide antibiotic.
Penicillin V Potassium	anti-infective antibiotic.
Amoxicillin	penicillin-like antibiotic.
Sulfisoxazole	sulfa antibiotic.

COMMON DRUGS

Trimethoprim / Sulfamethoxazole	sulfa antibiotic.
Tetracycline	bacteriostatic antibiotic.
Metronidazole	antibacterial and antiprotozoal agent.
Zidovudine	antiviral protease inhibitor.
Acyclovir	antiviral.
Nystatin	fungicidal, fungistatic agent.
Fluconazole	antifungal

ANTINEOPLASTICS

Cyclophosphamide	alkylating agent.
Cisplatin	alkylating agent.
Busulfan	alkylating agent.
Methotrexate	antimetabolite.
5-Fluorouracil	antimetabolite.
Mercaptopurine	antimetabolite.
Vincristine	plant alkaloid.
Paclitaxel	plant alkaloid.
Etoposide	plant alkaloid.
Tamoxifen Citrate	anti-estrogen.

CARDIOVASCULAR AGENTS

Nitroglycerin	antianginal agent.
Nifedipine	antianginal calcium channel blocker.
Verapamil Hydrochloride	antianginal calcium channel blocker.
Isosorbide Mononitrate	vasodilator.
Bretylium Tosylate	antiarrhythmic.
Lidocaine Hydrochloride	antiarrhythmic.
Diltiazem Hydrochloride	antihypertensive calcium channel blocker.
Doxazosin Mesylate	antihypertensive.
Losartan Potassium	antihypertensive.
Losartan / Hydrochlorothiazide	combination antihypertensive diuretic.
Amlodipine Besylate	antihypertensive calcium channel blocker.
Felodipine	antihypertensive calcium channel blocker.
Metaprolol Tartrate	antihypertensive beta blocker.
Furosemide	diuretic.
Benazepril Hydrochloride	antihypertensive ACE inhibitor.
Bisoprolol / Hydrochlorothiazide	combination antihypertensive beta blocker and diuretic.
Atenolol	antihypertensive beta blocker.
Terazosin Hydrochloride	antihypertensive.
Lisinopril	antihypertensive ACE inhibitor.
Hydrochlorothiazide	diuretic.

COMMON DRUGS

Dobutamine Hydrochloride	diuretic.
Dopamine Hydrochloride	diuretic.
Lovastatin	antihyperlipidemic.
Atorvastatin Calcium	antihyperlipidemic.
Simvastatin	antihyperlipidemic.
Fluvastatin Sodium	antihyperlipidemic.
Pravastatin Sodium	antihyperlipidemic.
Alteplase	thrombolytic.
Warfarin Sodium	anticoagulant.
Heparin	anticoagulant.

DERMATOLOGICALS

Hydrocortisone Cream	steroidal cream
Diphenhydramine Hydrochloride	antihistamine.
Silver Sulfadiazine	topical sulfa antibiotic.
Doxycycline Hyclate	tetracycline group antibiotic.
Clotrimazole / Betamethasone	topical antifungal and steroid.
Ofloxacin	broad spectrum antibiotic.

ELECTROLYTIC AGENTS

Potassium Chloride	potassium replacement
Sodium Chloride	salt replacement
Calcium Chloride	mineral
Magnesium Chloride	mineral

GASTROINTESTINAL AGENTS

Pancrelipase	pancreatic enzyme.
Loperamide Hydrochloride	antidiarrheal.
Diphenoxylate / Atropine	antidiarrheal.
Trimethobenzamide Hydrochloride	antiemetic.
Prochlorperazine Maleate	antiemetic.
Cimetidine	antacid, antiulcer.
Famotidine	antacid, antiulcer.
Lansoprazole	antacid, antiulcer.
Nizatidine	antacid, antiulcer.
Ranatidine Hydrochloride	antacid, antiulcer.
Cisapride	antacid, antiulcer.
Omeprazole	antacid, antiulcer.
Lactulose	laxative.
Docusate Sodium	stool softener.

Common Drugs

Hematological Agents

Desmopressin Acetate	coagulation enhancer.
Phytonadione	coagulation enhancer.
Ferrous Sulfate	hematopoietic.
Cyanocobalamin	hematopoietic.
Aminocaproic Acid	hemostatic agent.
Thrombin Powder	hemostatic agent.

Hormones & Modifiers

Fludrocortisone	adrenal agent.
Epinephrine	adrenal agent.
Glyburide	oral antidiabetic.
Glucagon	antidiabetic.
Insulin	antidiabetic.
Troglitazone	oral antidiabetic.
Glipizide	oral antihyperglycemic.
Metformin Hydrochloride	oral antidiabetic.
Glimepride	oral antihyperglycemic.
Methimazole	antithyroid agent.
Levothyroxine Sodium	synthetic thyroid hormone.
Calcitonin-Salmon	synthetic calcitonin.
Norethindrone / Ethinyl Estradiol	oral contraceptive.
Norethindrone / Mestranol	oral contraceptive.
Fluoxymesterone	androgen.
Sildenafil Citrate	erectile dysfunction agent.
Oxytocin	uterine contraction stimulant.
Clomiphene Citrate	fertility agent

Immunobiologic Agents

Diptheria Antitoxin	Diphtheria agent.
Immune Globulin	Hepatitis A, Rubeola, Varicella agent.
Hepatitis B Immune Globulin	Hepatitis B agent.
Rabies Immune Globulin	Rabies agent.
Tetanus Immune Globulin	Tetanus immunization agent.

Musculoskeletal Agents

Gold Sodium Thiomalate	rheumatoid arthritis agent.
Colchicine	anti-inflammatory.
Allopurinol	anti-gout.
Carisoprodol	muscle pain relief agent.
Cyclobenzaprine Hydrochloride	muscle antispasmodic and pain relief.
Diazepam	antispasmodic, antianxiety.

COMMON DRUGS

NEUROLOGICAL AGENTS

Carbidopa / Levodopa	anti-Parkinson's agent.
Benztropine Mesylate	anti-Parkinson's agent.
Tacrine Hydrochloride	anti-Alzheimer's.
Gabapentin	antiepileptic.
Phenytoin Sodium	antiepileptic.
Phenobarbital	barbiturate antiepileptic.
Ergotamine / Caffeine	antimigraine.
Sumatriptan Succinate	antimigraine.

OPHTHALMIC AGENTS

Physostigmine Sulfate	anti-glaucoma agent.
Betaxolol Hydrochloride	anti-glaucoma agent.
Timolol Maleate	anti-glaucoma agent.
Dipivefrin Hydrochloride	anti-glaucoma agent.
Gentamicin Sulfate	antibiotic.
Dexamethasone / Tobramycin	combination steroid and antibiotic.
Prednisolone Acetate	steroid.
Ketoralac Tromethamine	NSAID.

PSYCHOTROPIC AGENTS

Carbamazepine	mood stabilizer, anticonvulsant.
Divalproex Sodium	antidepressant, antianxiety, anticonvulsant.
Diazepam	antianxiety.
Lorazepam	antianxiety, sedative.
Alprazolam	antianxiety.
Buspirone Hydrochloride	antianxiety.
Paroxetine Hydrochloride	antidepressant SSRI.
Sertraline Hydrochloride	antidepressant SSRI.
Fluoxetine Hydrochloride	antidepressant SSRI.
Amitriptyline Hydrochloride	tricyclic antidepressant, sedative, pain relief.
Trazodone Hydrochloride	antidepressant.
Bupropion Hydrochloride	antidepressant.
Olanzapine	antipsychotic.
Chlorpromazine Hydrochloride	antipsychotic.
Trifluoperazine Hydrochloride	antipsychotic.
Haloperidol	antipsychotic.
Risperidone	antipsychotic.
Zolpidem Tartrate	hypnotic.
Disulfiram	alcohol aversion agent.
Naltrexone Hydrochloride	alcohol and narcotic addiction therapy.

RESPIRATORY AGENTS

COMMON DRUGS

Diphenhydramine Hydrochloride	antihistamine.
Fexofenadine Hydrochloride	antihistamine.
Loratidine	long acting antihistamine.
Cetirizine Hydrochloride	antihistamine.
Pseudoephedrine Hydrochloride	decongestant.
Phenylephrine Hydrochloride	decongestant.
Codeine / Guaifenesin	antitussive.
Benzonatate	antitussive.
Dextromethorphan	antitussive.
Acetylcysteine	mucolytic.
Guaifenesin	expectorant.
Metaproterenol Sulfate	bronchodilator.
Ipratropium Bromide	bronchodilator.
Albuterol Sulfate	bronchodilator.
Salmeterol Xinofoate	bronchodilator.
Theophylline	bronchodilator.
Triamcinolone Acetonide	anti-inflammatory.
Beclomethasone Dipropionate	anti-inflammatory.
Fluticasone Propionate	anti-inflammatory.

STUDY TIP — DRUG CARDS

A good way to help you remember the most common drugs used in pharmacy is to create drug cards. Drug cards are easy to make by writing the information from the previous list on small index cards. You can then use these to study until you have memorized the information.

Information needed on your drug card:

1. Trade name of drug

2. Generic name of drug

3. Main indication
   Note: Many drugs have more than one indication. You need to know only the main indication.

169

KEY CONCEPTS

Test your knowledge by covering the information in the right hand column.

USAN	The United States Adopted Names Council (USAN) designates nonproprietary names for drugs.
drug classes	Group names for drugs that have similar activities or are used for the same type of diseases and disorders.
stems	Common stems or syllables that are used to identify the different drug classes and in making new nonproprietary names. They are approved and recommended by the USAN.
neurotransmitter	Substances that carry the impulses from one neuron to another.
blocker	Another name for an antagonist drug -- because antagonists block the action of a neurotransmitter.
homeostasis	The state of equilibrium of the body.
mimetic	Another term for an agonist drug -- because agonists imitate or "mimic" the action of the neurotransmitter.
Lookalike/Soundalike	It is important to recognize that a number of drugs have similar sounding or looking names, but very different properties.
analgesia	A state in which pain is not felt even though a painful condition exists.
anti-pyretic	Reduces fever.
opiate-type analgesics	Drugs related to morphine and codeine that can be habit-forming and are used for pain relief.
narcotic analgesics	Same as opiate-type analgesics.
salicylates	Drugs related to aspirin that are used to relieve mild to moderate pain, and have anti-inflammatory and antipyretic properties.
NSAIDs	Non-steroidal anti-inflammatory drugs that have anti-inflammatory, antipyretic, and analgesic properties.
acetaminophen	A drug that relieves mild to moderate pain and has antipyretic properties.
local anesthetics	Drugs that block pain conduction from peripheral nerves to the central nervous system without causing a loss of consciousness.
surgical anesthesia	The stage of anesthesia in which surgery can be safely conducted.

medullary paralysis	An overdose of anesthesia that paralyzes the respiratory and heart centers of the medulla, leading to death.
antibiotic (antimicrobial)	Drug that destroys microorganisms.
antiviral	Drug that attacks a virus.
antifungal	Drug that destroys fungi or inhibits growth of fungi.
antimycobacterial	Drug that attacks the organisms that cause tuberculosis and leprosy.
antiprotozoal	Drug that destroys protozoa.
antihelminthic	Drug that destroys worms.
bactericidal	Bacteria killing.
bacteriostatic	Bacteria inhibiting.
virustatic	Drug that inhibits the growth of viruses.
antineoplastic	Drug that inhibits new growth of cancer cells.
lymphocyte	A type of white blood cell that releases antibodies that destroy disease cells.
metastasis	When cancer cells spread beyond their original site.
neoplasm	A new and abnormal tissue growth, often referring to cancer cells.
remission	A state in which cancer cells are inactive.
arrhythmia	An abnormal heart rhythm.
cardiac cycle	The contraction and relaxation of the heart that pumps blood through the cardiovascular system.
diastolic pressure	The minimum blood pressure when the heart relaxes; the second number in a blood pressure reading.
Electrocardiogram (EKG or ECG)	A graph of the heart's rhythm.
embolism	A clot that has traveled in the bloodstream to a point where it obstructs flow.
myocardium	Heart muscle.
systolic pressure	The maximum blood pressure when the heart contracts; the first number in a blood pressure reading.
thrombus	A blood clot.
antianginals	Drugs used to treat cardiac related chest pain (angina).

KEY CONCEPTS

Test your knowledge by covering the information in the right hand column.

antiarrhythmics	Drugs used to treat irregular heart rhythms.
antihypertensives	Drugs used to reduce a sustained elevation in blood pressure.
vasopressors	Drugs used to increase blood pressure.
antihyperlipidemics	Drugs used to lower high levels of cholesterol.
thrombolytics	Drugs used to dissolve blood clots.
anticoagulants	Drugs used to prevent blood clot formation.
beta blockers	Drugs that reduce the oxygen demands of the heart muscle.
calcium channel blockers	Drugs that relax the heart by reducing heart conduction.
diuretics	Drugs that decrease blood pressure by decreasing blood volume.
ACE inhibitors	The "pril" drugs that relax the blood vessels.
vasodilators	Drugs that relax and expand the blood vessels.
dermatological	A product that is used to treat a skin condition.
integumentary system	The skin.
anion	A negatively charged ion.
cation	A positively charged ion.
dissociation	When a compound breaks down and separates into smaller components.
electrolytes	A substance that in solution forms ions that conduct an electrical current.
extracellular fluids	The fluid outside the body's individual cells found in plasma and tissue fluid.
intracellular fluids	Cell fluid.
interstitial fluid	Tissue fluid.
ions	Electrically charged particles.
vaccine	A suspension containing infectious agents used to boost the body's immune system response.
chime	The semi-liquid form of food as it enters the intestinal tract.
peristalsis	The wave like motion of the intestines that moves food through them.

enzymes	Substances in the body that help the body to break down molecules.
antidiarrheals	Drugs used to treat diarrhea.
antiemetics	Drugs used to treat nausea and vomiting.
antacids	Drugs used to neutralize acid.
laxatives	Drugs that promote defecation.
stool softeners	Drugs that promote mixing of fatty and watery internal substances to soften the stool's contents and ease the evacuation of feces.
hematological agents	Drugs that affect the blood.
fibrin	The fiber that serves as the structure for clot formation.
anemia	A decrease in hemoglobin or red blood cells.
hemostatic drugs	Drugs that prevent excessive bleeding.
hormones	Chemicals that are secreted in the body by the endocrine system's ductless glands.
corticosteroid	Hormonal steroid substances produced by the cortex of the adrenal gland.
endocrine system	The system of hormone secreting glands.
hyperthyroidism	Overproduction of thyroid hormone.
hypothyroidism	Underproduction of thyroid hormone.
insulin	A hormone that controls the body's use of glucose.
glucagon	A hormone that helps convert amino acid to glucose.
diabetes mellitus	A condition in which the body does not produce enough insulin or is unable to use insulin efficiently.
serum glucose	Blood sugar.
androgens	Male sex hormones.
estrogen	Female sex characteristic hormone that is involved in calcium and phosphorus conservation.
progesterone	Female sex characteristic hormone that is involved in ovulation prevention.
testosterone	The primary androgen (male sex hormone).
gout	A painful inflammatory condition in which excess uric acid accumulates in the joints.

KEY CONCEPTS

Test your knowledge by covering the information in the right hand column.

rheumatoid arthritis	A chronic and often progressive inflammatory condition with symptoms that include swelling, feelings of warmth, and joint pain.
osteoarthritis	A disorder characterized by weight-bearing bone deterioration, decreasing range of motion, pain, and deformity.
Parkinson's Disease	A progressive neuromuscular condition.
Alzheimer's Disease	A progressive dementia condition.
epilepsy	A neurologic disorder characterized by seizures.
migraine headaches	A type of headache associated with possible auras and pain.
ophthalmic agents	Drugs used to treat conditions of the eye.
conjunctivitis	Inflammation of the eyelid lining.
glaucoma	A disorder characterized by high pressure within the eye.
mydriatics	Drugs that dilate the pupil.
sedatives	Drugs that are intended to relax and calm.
hypnotics	Drugs that are intended to induce sleep.
bipolar disorder	A disorder characterized by mood swings.
depression	A disorder characterized by low mood.
asthma	A condition characterized by chronic airway inflammation.
emphysema	A condition associated with chronic airway obstruction.
antihistamines	Drugs that replace histamine at histamine receptor sites.
decongestants	Drugs that cause mucous membrane vasoconstriction.
antitussives	Drugs that are used to treat coughs.
bronchodilators	Drugs that are used to relieve bronchospasm.

STUDY NOTES

Use this area to write important points you'd like to remember.

FILL IN THE BLANKS

Match the drug classifications with the generic drug names. Answers are at the end of the book.

Analgesic	Antineoplastic	Gastrointestinal Agent
Anesthetic	Cardiovascular Agent	Musculoskeletal Agent
Antidiabetic	Dermatological Agent	Respiratory Agent
Anti-infective	Electrolytic Agent	

Generic Name   **Drug Classification**

1. Acetaminophen _____

2. Albuterol _____

3. Amlodipine _____

4. Amoxicillin / Clavulanate _____

5. Ampicillin _____

6. Aspirin _____

7. Atenolol _____

8. Azithromycin _____

9. Carisoprodol _____

10. Cefaclor _____

11. Cimetidine _____

12. Ciprofloxacin _____

13. Clarithromycin _____

14. Clotrimazole/Betamethazone _____

15. Cyclophosphamide _____

16. Diltiazem _____

17. Docusate Sodium _____

18. Doxazosin _____

19. Fluconazole _____

20. Furosemide _____

21. Glyburide _____

22. Heparin _____

23. Hydrocortisone Cream _____

24. Ibuprofen _____

25. Insulin _____

26. Ipratorpium _____

27. Lactulose _____

28. Lansoprazole _____

29. Loperamide _____

30. Losartan _____

31. Lovastatin _____

32. Metaprolol _____

33. Nifedipine _____

34. Nitroglycerin _____

35. Nitrous oxide _____

36. Nizatidine _____

37. Omeprazole _____

38. Potassium Chloride _____

39. Propoxyphene _____

40. Silver Sulfadiazine _____

41. Sodium Chloride _____

42. Tamoxifen _____

43. Tetracaine _____

44. Tramadol _____

45. Trimethobenzamide _____

46. Trimethoprim/Sulfamethoxazole _____

47. Verapamil _____

48. Warfarin _____

PRACTICE EXAM

The following multiple choice questions are in the *choose the best answer format* of the National Pharmacy Technician Certification Examination. There are four possible answers with only one answer being the most correct. Many of these questions can be answered through a careful review of this workbook. However, others require knowledge gained from practice as a technician. Answers for all questions can be found at the end of the exam.

Since the time limit for taking the National Exam is three hours, you may want to test your ability to answer the questions under a time limit, or you may simply wish to time yourself to see how long it takes you. There are 140 questions here, the same number as on the exam. If you wish to have a similar experience, you can allow yourself three hours to answer these questions.

For more information on the National Exam, see the preface of this Workbook.

Answers are on page 214.

1. The pharmacist has asked you to obtain a MedWatch form so s/he can report

   a. an adverse event regarding a veterinary product.
   b. an adverse event regarding a drug.
   c. an adverse event regarding a vaccine.
   d. an adverse event regarding a medical device.

2. Medications for ophthalmic administration are usually available in _____ or _____.

   a. sterile hypotonic drops or sterile ointment
   b. sterile hypertonic drops or sterile ointment
   c. hypotonic solution or hypotonic suspension
   d. sterile isotonic drops or sterile ointment

3. A Class _____ drug recall is the most serious.

   a. I
   b. II
   c. III
   d. IV

4. Most drugs are metabolized by the

   a. liver.
   b. kidneys.
   c. gall bladder.
   d. gastrointestinal tract.

5. Nolvadex® or _____ is an anti-estrogen type medication that is often used in the treatment of breast cancer.

   a. albuterol
   b. tamoxifen
   c. phenytoin
   d. nifedipine

6. Tylenol No. 3 is acetaminophen 325 mg and codeine _____mg.

   a. 15 mg
   b. 30 mg
   c. 60 mg
   d. none of the above

Answers are on page 214.

7. When using a Class A prescription balance, the least weighable quantity is

   a. 6 mg.
   b. 120 mg.
   c. 500 mg.
   d. the same as the sensitivity requirement.

8. The form number for ordering Schedule II drugs is

   a. DEA Form 121.
   b. DEA Form 200.
   c. DEA Form 222.
   d. DEA Form 240.

9. Which drug can be used as a patch?

   a. nupercainal ointment
   b. clonidine
   c. amoxicillin
   d. vitamin C

10. How much diluent do you need to add to a 4 gm vial to get a concentration of 250 mg / ml? Disregard the space the powder may occupy.

    a. 12 ml
    b. 14 ml
    c. 16 ml
    d. 18 ml

11. The smallest gelatin capsule used for extemporaneous compounding is size

    a. 10.
    b. 8.
    c. 5.
    d. 000.

12. Which type of drug would be considered a drug of abuse?

    a. opiates
    b. alcohol
    c. nicotine
    d. all of the above

Answers are on page 214.

13. Furosemide or Lasix® is used as

    a. an analgesic.
    b. an anti-inflammatory agent.
    c. a sedative.
    d. a diuretic.

14. The infusion rate of an IV is over 12 hours. The total exact volume is 800 ml. What would be the infusion rate in mls per minute?

    a. 0.56 ml / minute
    b. 1.11 ml / minute
    c. 2.7 ml / minute
    d. none of the above

15. You have a 70% solution of dextrose. How many grams of dextrose is in 400 ml of this solution?

    a. 700 grams
    b. 460 grams
    c. 280 grams
    d. 120 grams

16. The standard pediatric dose for cefazolin is 20 mg/kg/day. The order is written for 150 mg TID. The infant weighs 8 lb. This dose is

    a. too high.
    b. too low.
    c. within guidelines.

17. Federal law requires pharmacies to have available for inspection Copy 3 of the DEA Form 222 for a period of _____ year(s).

    a. 1
    b. 4
    c. 3
    d. 2

18. An IV order calls for the addition of 45 mEq of $CaCO_3$ (calcium carbonate). You have a 25 ml vial of $CaCO_3$ 4.4mEq/ml. How many mls of this concentrate do you need to add to this IV?

    a. 5.6 ml
    b. 8.4 ml
    c. 10.2 ml
    d. 12.8 ml

Answers are on page 214.

19. In this formula, how much talc is needed to fill 120 grams?

    nupercainal ointment   4%

    zinc oxide   20%

    talc   2%

    a. 1200 mg
    b. 1500 mg
    c. 2000 mg
    d. 2400 mg

20. A bottle of nitroglycerin has the labeled strength of 1/200 grains. What would this strength be in milligrams?

    a. 0.2 mg
    b. 0.3 mg
    c. 0.4 mg
    d. 0.6 mg

21. A pharmacy wants to mark-up a product by thirty percent. How much would an item cost with this mark-up, if its original cost was $4.50?

    a. $5.85
    b. $6.23
    c. $6.40
    d. $7.10

22. The _____ is the agency that registers pharmacists.

    a. Department of Public Health
    b. NAPLEX
    c. Joint Commission
    d. State Board of Pharmacy

23. The Material Safety Data Sheets (MSDS)

    a. provide protocols for fire hazards in the pharmacy setting.
    b. provide safety codes by OSHA in the storage of inventory.
    c. provide information concerning hazardous substances.
    d. none of the above.

Answers are on page 214.

24. How much diluent do you need to add to 4 gm of powder to get a concentration of 500 mg/ml?

   a. 0.8 ml
   b. 8 ml
   c. 1.0 ml
   d. 10 ml

25. What does DAW mean on a written prescription?

   a. the medication ordered is a controlled substance
   b. the medication should be taken with water
   c. the brand name is to be dispensed as written
   d. refills are limited to six months

26. Your pharmacy has received a prescription for Ointment XYZ and is not available commercially. The prescription is written for 30 g with 2 refills. According to FDA guidelines, what is the largest amount your pharmacy can compound when originally filling the prescription in anticipation of refills?

   a. 90 g
   b. 120 g
   c. 30 g
   d. 60 g

27. The last set of digits of the NDC are indicative of

   a. the manufacturer.
   b. product identification.
   c. package size.
   d. none of the above.

28. The approximate size container for the dispensing of 180 ml of liquid medication would be?

   a.) 2 ounces
   b.) 4 ounces
   c.) 6 ounces
   d.) 8 ounces

Answers are at on page 214.

29. A patient asks whether he/she can take a certain medication with another one? As a pharmacy technician what should you do?

    a. inform the patient that you see no problem
    b. provide the patient with a drug insert
    c. request the patient see the pharmacist for a consult
    d. try to sell the patient some Mylanta®

30. The doctor writes: ii gtts OU bid. What does this mean?

    a. two drops in the left eye twice a day
    b. two drops in the right eye twice a day
    c. two drops in each eye twice a day
    d. two drops in the right ear twice a day

31. Which of the following suppositories should be stored in the refrigerator?

    a. Phenergan®
    b. Thorazine®
    c. Tigan®
    d. Compazine®

32. Which of the following books is used for FDAs list of approved drug products?

    a. Merck Index
    b. Red Book
    c. Orange Book
    d. Martindale

33. Propranolol is the same as

    a. Inderal.
    b. Tenormin.
    c. lisinopril.
    d. Corgard.

34. Thiazide diuretics are used to

    a. relieve migraine headaches.
    b. relieve gastroenteritis.
    c. manage of pain.
    d. manage the retention of water.

Answers are on page 214.

35. Of the following, which one deals with the issue of safety caps on prescription bottles?

    a. The Controlled Substance Act
    b. The Poison Prevention Act
    c. Hazardous Substance Act
    d. Federal Food and Cosmetic Act

36. An example of a major drug-drug interaction would be

    a. warfarin-aspirin.
    b. digoxin-diltiazem.
    c. penicillin-cephalosporin.
    d. hydrocodone-codeine.

37. The appearance of crystals in mannitol injection would indicate that the product

    a. was exposed to cold.
    b. has settled during shipment.
    c. contains impurities and should be returned.
    d. was formulated using sterile saline.

38. How many 30 mg $KMNO_4$ (Potassium Permanganate) tablets are needed to make the following solution? $KMNO_4$ 1:5000 600 ml

    a. 2 tablets
    b. 3 tablets
    c. 4 tablets
    d. 6 tablets

39. Dextrose 25% 1000ml is ordered. You have only dextrose 70% solution available. How much of the dextrose 70% solution and sterile water will you use to fill this order?

    a. 250 ml dextrose 70% and 750 ml sterile water
    b. 357 ml dextrose 70% and 643 ml sterile water
    c. 424 ml dextrose 70% and 576 ml sterile water
    d. none of the above

Answers are on page 214.

40. The Occupational, Safety, Health Administration (OSHA) requires pharmacies to have Material Safety Data Sheets (MSDS) for

    a. all drugs in the pharmacy inventory.
    b. all materials stored in the pharmacy refrigerator.
    c. each hazardous chemical used in the pharmacy.
    d. all controlled substances in the pharmacy inventory.

41. Of the following group names, which one would be used for cough?

    a. antihelmintics
    b. antitussives
    c. antihistamines
    d. anticholinergics

42. Tobrex® ophthalmic ung refers to

    a. an ointment used for the eye.
    b. a solution used for the eye.
    c. a topical ointment for external use only.
    d. an ointment used for the ear.

43. Suspending or thickening agents are added to suspensions to thicken the suspending medium and retard the sedimentation rate. Which of the following is not a suspending agent?

    a. carboxymethylcellulose
    b. tragacanth
    c. acacia
    d. bentonite

44. Oral Polio Virus Vaccine (Poliovax®) should be stored in a temperature not to exceed 46 degrees Fahrenheit. What is this temperature in Centigrade? Use this formula: Centigrade = 5/9 (F° - 32°)

    a. 6 degrees C
    b. 8 degrees C
    c. 10 degrees C
    d. 12 degrees C

Answers are on page 214.

45. You receive a prescription for amoxicillin 75 mg QID for ten days. How many mls of amoxicillin 250 mg /5ml do you need to fill this prescription to last the full ten days?

    a. 20 ml
    b. 40 ml
    c. 60 ml
    d. 100 ml

46. The doctor writes for aminophylline 125 mg po QID x 10 days. You only have the solution 250 mg/5 ml. How much would be needed for one dose?

    a. 1/4 teaspoonful
    b. 1/2 teaspoonful
    c. 3/4 teaspoonful
    d. 1 1/2 teaspoonful

47. Of the following schedules, which one deals with drugs that have no medicinal use in the United States and have a high abuse potential?

    a. Schedule I
    b. Schedule II
    c. Schedule III
    d. Schedule IV

48. You receive a prescription for sertraline (Zoloft®) qd x 30 days. What is sertraline?

    a. antihypertensive
    b. anticonvulsant
    c. antidepressant
    d. antianginal

49. All aseptic manipulations in the the laminar flow hood should be performed at least

    a. four inches within the hood.
    b. six inches within the hood.
    c. eight inches within the hood.
    d. twelve inches within the hood.

PRACTICE EXAM

Answers are on page 214.

50. Pharmacy technicians can perform their duties provided they

    a. check everything they do.
    b. read all labels three times.
    c. have all labels and products checked by a Pharmacist.
    d. are certified.

51. You receive an order for kaopectate 30 ml bid prn. How many tablespoonsful is one dose equal to?

    a. 5 tablespoons
    b. 3 tablespoons
    c. 2 tablespoons
    d. 1 tablespoon

52. Which of the following is a Schedule II Controlled Substance?

    a. diazepam
    b. meperidine
    c. pentazocine
    d. propoxyphene

53. If the manufacturer's expiration date for a drug is 12/06, the drug is considered acceptable to dispense until which date?

    a. 12/01/06
    b. 12/31/06
    c. 11/30/06
    d. 1/01/07

54. The Roman numerals XLII is equivalent to

    a. 42.
    b. 62.
    c. 92.
    d. 402.

55. A small volume intravenous bag specifically used to deliver medication is called an

    a. IV.
    b. IVPB.
    c. injection.
    d. none of the above.

Answers are on page 214.

56. How many days will the following prescription last?
    Prozac® 10mg #120   *Sig: 2 po BID*

    a. 20 days
    b. 30 days
    c. 45 days
    d. 60 days

57. The laminar flow hood should be left operating continuously. If it is turned off, it should not be used until it has been running for at least

    a. ten minutes.
    b. thirty minutes.
    c. forty-five minutes.
    d. sixty minutes.

58. Which auxiliary label would you use for this particular sig: ii gtts AU bid?

    a. take with meals
    b. for the ear
    c. avoid sunlight
    d. for the eye

59. A dose is written for 5 mg/kg every eight hours for one day. The adult to take this medication weighs 145 pounds. How much drug will be needed to fill this order?

    a. 765 mg
    b. 844 mg
    c. 989 mg
    d. 1254 mg

60. How much medication would be needed for the following order?
    prednisone 10 mg, one qid x 4 days, one tid x 2 days, one bid x 1 day, then stop

    a. 16
    b. 20
    c. 24
    d. 26

61. Benzethidine is in DEA Schedule I, meaning that benzethidine

    a. has a currently accepted medical use in the United States with severe restrictions.
    b. can only be handled by the pharmacist.
    c. has no currently accepted medical use in the world.
    d. has no currently accepted medical use in the United States.

PRACTICE EXAM

Answers are on page 214.

62. In which controlled substance schedule is Tylenol® No. 2 classified?

    a. Schedule I
    b. Schedule II
    c. Schedule III
    d. Schedule IV

63. Assuming that one pint is equal to 473 ml, how many pints can be found in one liter?

    a. 1.5 pints
    b. 2.1 pints
    c. 2.8 pints
    d. 3.1 pints

64. Licensing and general professional oversight of pharmacists and pharmacies are carried out by

    a. colleges of pharmacy.
    b. state board of pharmacy.
    c. the American Pharmaceutical Association.
    d. the United States Pharmacopeial Convention.

65. Most unit-dose systems provide each patient with a storage bin in which can be found a supply of drugs for

    a. six hours.
    b. eight hours.
    c. twenty-four hours.
    d. forty-eight hours.

66. The first line of defense against infection/contamination of an IV product is

    a. antibiotics.
    b. antiseptics.
    c. disinfectants.
    d. handwashing.

67. The most widely used reference of an IV admixture program is (the)

    a. Handbook of Injectable Drugs.
    b. Redbook.
    c. Remington's.
    d. Martindale's.

Answers are on page 214.

68. Which of the following medications must be administered in a glass IV container?

    a. aminophylline
    b. dopamine
    c. nitroglycerin
    d. potassium

69. Preservative-free drugs must be used when drugs will be injected by which route of administration?

    a. intramuscular
    b. intrathecal
    c. intravenous
    d. subcutaneous

70. The two parts of the syringe that should not be touched are

    a. the tip and collar.
    b. the collar and barrel
    c. the tip and plunger.
    d. the collar and plunger.

71. The establishment of the Omnibus Budget Reconciliation Act (OBRA) in 1990, led to most states requiring

    a. the use of pharmacy technicians.
    b. the counseling of patients by pharmacists.
    c. the enactment of the Controlled Substance Act.
    d. inventory management of each pharmacy setting.

72. The first five digits of the National Drug Code (NDC) number identifies the

    a. product.
    b. manufacturer.
    c. units.
    d. type of packaging.

73. Sig or signa on a written prescription means

    a. the strength of the medication ordered.
    b. the quantity of medication ordered.
    c. the directions for the medication ordered.
    d. the signature of the Practitioner writing the medication ordered.

Answers are at the end of the exam.

74. From the following directions how many tablets should be dispensed?
2 tabs po qid x 2 days, then 1 tab po tid x 2 days, then ss po bid x 2 days, then dc

    a. 22
    b. 23
    c. 24
    d. none of the above

75. What should the last digit be of this DEA number?
AB431762 __

    a. one
    b. three
    c. five
    d. seven

76. Aminosyn is an amino acid often used in TPN orders to provide protein for cellular repair and growth. A physician writes an order for aminosyn 2.5% 500 ml. You have only aminosyn 8.5% 500 ml. How are you going to prepare this order using a sterile evacuated container?

    a. add 320 ml of aminosyn 8.5% and qs with sterile water to 500 ml
    b. add 147 ml of aminosyn 8.5% and qs with sterile water to 500 ml
    c. add 124 ml of aminosyn 8.5% and qs with sterile water to 500 ml
    d. add 74 ml of aminosyn 8.5% and qs with sterile water to 500 ml

77. You are to use 2.4 ml of diluent to reconstitute a vial of medication. What size of syringe should be used?

    a. 20 ml
    b. 10 ml
    c. 5 ml
    d. 3 ml

78. The use of isopropyl alcohol is important as a means to prevent contamination of an IV product. What should the minimum percent of isopropyl alcohol used be?

    a. 50%
    b. 70%
    c. 90%
    d. 100%

Answers are at the end of the exam.

79. Most drugs and their metabolites are excreted by the

    a. liver.
    b. kidneys.
    c. gall bladder.
    d. gastrointestinal tract.

80. The percentage or fraction of the administered dose of a drug that actually reaches systemic circulation and the rate at which this occurs is the drugs

    a. bioequivalence.
    b. bioavailability.
    c. biotransformation.
    d. therapeutic equivalence.

81. The type of formulary that allows the pharmacy to obtain all medications that are prescribed is a(an)

    a. international formulary.
    b. closed formulary.
    c. wholesaler formulary.
    d. open formulary.

82. Zantac, Tagamet and Pepcid are H_2 blockers which are now available over-the-counter (OTC). What are these drugs used for?

    a. used as an antihistamine to alleviate runny nose
    b. used as an decongestant to unclog nasal passages
    c. used to inhibit stomach acid secretion
    d. used as an antacid in that it neutralizes stomach acid

83. A "hospital borne" infection is also known as a _____ infection.

    a. nosocomial
    b. infectious
    c. superinfection
    d. none of the above

84. Of the following drug recalls, which one is the most important in that all parties involved in the dispensing of a prescription (doctor, pharmacy and patient) must be notified due to the drugs potential or serious harm?

    a. Drug Recall I
    b. Drug Recall II
    c. Drug Recall III
    d. Drug Recall IV

Answers are on page 214.

85. Reconstitution with Ampicillin (Omnipen®) IVPB should be done with

    a. D5% Water.
    b. 0.9% NaCl.
    c. tap water.
    d. vinegar.

86. A prescription for amoxicillin 250 mg #30 has a usual and customary price of $8.49. The acquisition cost of amoxicillin 250mg #30 is $2.02. What is the gross profit?

    a. $2.02
    b. $6.47
    c. 50%
    d. 1/3

87. A senior citizen is paying for a prescription for penicillin VK 250 mg #30. The usual and customary price is $8.49. However this patient qualifies for a 10% discount. How much will the patient pay?

    a. $8.49
    b. $6.99
    c. $8.39
    d. $7.64

88. NPH U-100 insulin contains 100 units of insulin per ml. The AWP for one 10 ml bottle of it is $18.45. The acquisition cost to the pharmacy for a 10 ml bottle is $16.70. The usual and customary price for one bottle of NPH U-100 insulin at that pharmacy is $14.99. If the pharmacy has an agreement with the third-party plan for reimbursement of 87% AWP or 100% U&C (whichever is less) + a $3.50 dispensing fee, what will be the total amount of the third-party claim?

    a. $18.49
    b. $19.55
    c. $20.20
    d. $21.95

89. A prescription is written for Septra Suspension 240 ml 1 teaspoonful h.s. + 1 refill. The insurance plan has a 34-day supply limitation. How many ml can be dispensed using the insurance plan guidelines?

    a. 120 ml
    b. 170 ml
    c. 240 ml
    d. 360 ml

Answers are on page 214.

90. A prescription is written for Albuterol Inhaler: Dispense 2 inhalers of 17 gm, 2 puffs q.i.d. What is the days supply if there are 200 metered doses in each inhaler?

    a. 34
    b. 50
    c. 25
    d. 20

91. A prescription is written for Humulin N U-100 insulin 10 ml, 40 units daily. What is the days supply?

    a. 25
    b. 34
    c. 21
    d. 28

92. A prescription is written for Tetracycline HCl suspension 125 mg/5 ml compounded from capsules and a mixture of Ora-Plus 50% and Ora-Sweet 50%. How many capsules of Tetracycline 250 mg are needed to prepare 50 ml of this suspension?

    a. 5
    b. 10
    c. 15
    d. 20

93. Convert the Celsius temperature of 100 degrees into degrees Fahrenheit.

    a. 132
    b. 68
    c. 212
    d. 0

94. How many doses are in a 100 ml bottle of penicillin VK 250 mg/5 ml if each dose is 1/2 teaspoonful?

    a. 10
    b. 20
    c. 30
    d. 40

Answers are on page 214.

95. More than 3/4 of sales from pharmaceutical manufacturers are directly to

    a. wholesalers.
    b. chain pharmacies.
    c. hospitals.
    d. mail order pharmacies.

96. How many teaspoons equal 20 ml?

    a. 5
    b. 6
    c. 4
    d. 2

97. If a prescription reads: Aspirin 5gr, dispense 100 tablets, 1 tablet q 4-6h prn headache, what is the dose in milligrams?

    a. 650
    b. 750
    c. 100
    d. 325

98. How many gallons of Coca Cola fountain syrup are needed to package 150 bottles of 120 ml per bottle?

    a. 3
    b. 4
    c. 5
    d. 6

99. If a prescription reads: Amoxicillin 250 mg/5 ml, dispense 150 ml, 375 mg t.i.d. x 5d, what is the dose in household units?

    a. 1 teaspoonful
    b. 1 tablespoonful
    c. 1.5 teaspoonful
    d. 1.5 tablespoonful

100. How many ml are in 2 liters of normal saline?

    a. 200
    b. 2,000
    c. 0.2
    d. 0.002

Answers are on page 214.

101. How many ml of KCl 2 mEq/ml are needed if the dose is 30 mEq?

    a. 5
    b. 10
    c. 15
    d. 30

102. How many ml of 25% dextrose are needed to prepare 500 ml of 40% dextrose if you are to prepare 40% dextrose from 25% dextrose and 60% dextrose?

    a. 214 ml
    b. 286 ml
    c. 200 ml
    d. 300 ml

103. If 1 liter is infused over 8 hours, what is the rate of infusion in ml/hr?

    a. 62.5
    b. 100
    c. 125
    d. 250

104. A patient weighs 121 pounds. What is the patient's weight in kg?

    a. 37
    b. 45
    c. 55
    d. 68

105. How many grams of sodium bicarbonate are needed to make 400 ml of a 1:1000 w/v solution?

    a. 0.2
    b. 0.4
    c. 0.8
    d. 1

106. Which of the following medications is associated with gradual discontinuation of therapy?

    a. Amoxil
    b. Sumycin
    c. Medrol
    d. Zovirax

PRACTICE EXAM

Answers are on page 214.

107. Alprozolam is a/an:

 a. narcotic
 b. barbiturate
 c. benzodiazepine
 d. stimulant

108. A medication to reduce fever is called a/an

 a. antitussive.
 b. antipyretic.
 c. expectorant.
 d. analgesic.

109. What medication may cause an allergic reaction if a patient is allergic to penicillin and Ceclor?

 a. zithromycin
 b. doxycycline
 c. cefaclor
 d. amantadine

110. A prescription for Duragesic patches should be filed under which DEA schedule?

 a. Schedule I
 b. Schedule II
 c. Schedule III
 d. Schedule IV

111. Which of the following medications is most likely to be associated with photosensitivity?

 a. Bactrim
 b. Amoxil
 c. Suprax
 d. Cleocin

112. A pharmacist should be alerted about possible drug interactions when _____ and _____ are prescribed for the same patient.

 a. Zantac and Zocor
 b. Allopurinol and ibuprofen
 c. Darvocet N-100 and Dyazide
 d. Coumadin and Percodan

Answers are on page 214.

113. Which of the following medications is classified in DEA Schedule III?

   a. Percodan
   b. Percocet
   c. Vicodin
   d. Valium

114. Which of the following medications is an antidiarrheal?

   a. propranolol
   b. famotidine
   c. methylphenidate
   d. loperamide

115. Vitamin A is a _____-soluble vitamin and Vitamin C is a _____-soluble vitamin.

   a. water, water
   b. fat, water
   c. fat, fat
   d. water, fat

116. Which of the following medications contains morphine?

   a. Demerol
   b. Dolophine
   c. MS Contin
   d. Mobigesic

117. If a medication is to be taken a.c., it should be taken

   a. in the morning.
   b. around the clock.
   c. after meals.
   d. before meals.

118. The federal agency associated with the Controlled Substances Act is the

   a. ASHP.
   b. DEA.
   c. Treasury Department.
   d. FDA.

Answers are on page 214.

119. The receipt of orders for Schedule III controlled substances can be documented on

    a. DEA Form 222.
    b. the invoice/packing slip from wholesaler
    c. DEA Form 600.
    d. FDA form 1210.

120. Which DEA number fails the numerical check for DEA numbers?

    a. AK 6782329
    b. AB 3081421
    c. AG 1355672
    d. BS 3421234

121. An example of an H2 receptor blocker is:

    a. Pepcid
    b. Lomotil
    c. Chlor-Trimeton
    d. Prilosec

122. The directions "ii gtt o.u. q.i.d." indicate the medication is a/an

    a. otic.
    b. ophthalmic.
    c. oral.
    d. ointment.

123. _____ is an example of an anabolic steroid.

    a. Methylprednisolone
    b. Prednisone
    c. Testosterone
    d. Conjugated estrogens

124. Vasotec is a member of which of the following classes of drugs?

    a. antibiotic
    b. beta-blocker
    c. calcium channel blocker
    d. ACE inhibitor

Answers are on page 214.

125. A pharmacist should be alerted if a patient is allergic to codeine and is prescribed

    a. Xanax.
    b. Klonopin.
    c. Tussi-Organidin.
    d. Ritalin.

126 A term used to describe the rate that inventory is used is

    a. MSDS.
    b. turnover.
    c. POS.
    d. spoilage.

127. Storing drugs a room temperature means storing at

    a. between 59 and 86 degrees F.
    b. between 65 and 75 degrees F.
    c. between 40 and 42 degrees F.
    d. less than 80 degrees F.

128. Child resistant caps are required for

    a. only for prescriptions intended for children.
    b. all prescriptions unless the patient requests an easy open cap.
    c. only for prescriptions dispensed to household with children.
    d. those prescriptions where a child resistant cap is required as determined by professional judgement.

129. The first federal drug law was the

    a. Food Drug and Cosmetic Act.
    b. Durham-Humphrey Amendment.
    c. Pure Food and Drugs Act.
    d. Kefauver-Harris Amendment.

130. HIPAA requires that

    a. all Medicaid patients are offered counseling by a pharmacist.
    b. all patients receive counseling by a pharmacist.
    c. all patients are offered counseling by a pharmacist.
    d. privacy rules are observed for protected health information.

PRACTICE EXAM
Answers are on page 214.

131. Nitroglycerin is available in a sublingual tablet. This means that

    a. the tablet should be dissolved in the cheek.
    b. the tablet should be swallowed whole.
    c. the medication can only be dispensed in a glass container.
    d. the tablet should be dissolved under the tongue.

132. The _____ is the most often used form for billing disease state management services.

    a. UCF
    b. online adjudication
    c. CMS-1500 (formerly HCFA 1500)
    d. Form 222

133. Membrane filters are intended to filer a solution

    a. from a suspension.
    b. as the solution is pulled into the syringe.
    c. as the solution is expelled from a syringe.
    d. as the needle is removed from the syringe.

134. For needles sizes, a higher gauge number means

    a. the syringe is smaller.
    b. the bevel is smaller.
    c. the lumen is smaller.
    d. the hub is smaller.

135. The resulting solution, when a drug is added to a parenteral solution is called

    a. lyophilized.
    b. an admixture.
    c. a lock.
    d. a diluent.

136. Licenses for controlled substances are issued by the

    a. JCAHO.
    b. APhA.
    c. State Board.
    d. DEA.

Answers on page 214.

137. The managed care network that covers costs inside, but not outside of the network is

   a. POS.
   b. HMO.
   c. PBM.
   d. PPO.

138. The federal-state program that provides health care for the needy is called

   a. PAP.
   b. Medicaid.
   c. Medicare.
   d. HMO.

139. When completing a universal claim form, drugs are billed using the

   a. UPIN.
   b. NDC.
   c. 222.
   d. CMS-1500 (formerly HCFA 1500).

140. The Orange Book provides information about

   a. investigational drugs.
   b. drug product stability.
   c. current pricing.
   d. generic equivalents.

CALCULATIONS PRACTICE EXAM

The following multiple choice problems provide you with extra practice with pharmacy calculations before taking the National Exam. There are four possible answers for each problem, with only one answer being the most correct. Similar to the questions in the Practice Exam, many of the problems in the Calculations Practice Exam can be solved using techniques that are included in this workbook; however, others require knowledge gained from practice as a technician.

Pharmacy calculations must be carefully done with 100% accuracy. Therefore, you should practice doing calculations using a systematic approach for problem-solving and always double-check your work. This Calculations Practice Exam contains 40 problems that are designed to provide you with extra practice with pharmacy calculations before taking the National Exam.

PRACTICE EXAM

Answers are on page 214.

1.   You are filling a prescription that reads: Amoxicillin 125 mg/5 ml, Sig 1 tsp t.i.d. Dispense 150 ml. How many milliliters should the patient take each day?

     a.   5 ml
     b.   10 ml
     c.   15 ml
     d.   20 ml

2.   You are filling a prescription that reads: EES 200, Sig 1 tsp t.i.d. Dispense 150 ml. How many days should this prescription last?

     a.   5 days
     b.   7 days
     c.   10 days
     d.   14 days

3.   A compounded prescription calls for 600 gm of white petrolatum. How many 1 lb jars should you obtain so there is enough to prepare this prescription?

     a.   1 jar
     b.   2 jars
     c.   3 jars
     d.   4 jars

4.   Each tablet of Tylenol #3 has 30 mg of codeine. How many grains of codeine are in each tablet of Tylenol #3?

     a.   1/2 grain
     b.   1 grain
     c.   2 grains
     d.   3 grains

5.   One form of influenza vaccine, the Live Attenuated Intranasal Vaccine, must be stored at -15 degrees C. What is this temperature in degrees F?

     a.   5 degrees F
     b.   -5 degrees F
     c.   27 degrees F
     d.   -27 degrees F

CALCULATIONS PRACTICE EXAM

Answers are on page 214.

6. The lead pharmacy technician must reorder billing forms when 80% of the case has been used. A full case of billing forms contains 20 packages of forms. How many packages of forms should be remaining in the case when it's time to reorder?

    a. 16 packages
    b. 12 packages
    c. 8 packages
    d. 4 packages

7. In reconstituting a liquid antibiotic, 90 ml of distilled water should be used. If 1/3 of the water should be added first to moisten the powder, how much water should be added to moisten the powder?

    a. 45 ml
    b. 60 ml
    c. 15 ml
    d. 30 ml

8. How many capsules of clindamycin hydrochloride should be used to prepare 30 ml of the following preparation, if each capsule contains 150 mg of clindamycin hydrochloride?
        clindamycin hydrochloride   600 mg
        70% isopropyl alcohol   qs ad 60 ml

    a. 4 capsules
    b. 2 capsules
    c. 10 capsules
    d. 20 capsules

9. A prescription is written for ibuprofen 10% cream. How much ibuprofen is needed to make 20 gm of the cream?

    a. 400 mg
    b. 200 mg
    c. 2 gm
    d. 4 gm

10. You are entering a prescription for an albuterol inhaler that delivers 90 mcg per actuation. If each container delivers 200 actuations and each dose is two actuations, how many mg are delivered in each dose?

    a. 180 mg
    b. 90 mg
    c. 0.18 mg
    d. 0.09 mg

Answers are on page 214.

11. What is the days supply for a Z-Pak that contains six azithromycin 250 mg tablets, with directions of 500 mg on the first day, followed by 250 mg once daily until gone?

    a. 3
    b. 5
    c. 4
    d. 6

12. What is the da's supply for metronidazole vaginal gel 70 g, Sig 5 g twice daily?

    a. 5 days
    b. 7 days
    c. 10 days
    d. 14 days

13. What is the days supply for Humulin N insulin 20 ml, if the dose is 40 U daily?

    a. 100 days
    b. 30 days
    c. 60 days
    d. 50 days

14. How much change should be given to a patient who gives you $50 to pay for 3 prescriptions if the patient's prescription plan has a $10 copay?

    a. $20
    b. $10
    c. $40
    d. $30

15. What is the gross profit for a prescription if the selling price is $73.14, the acquisition cost is $52.10, and the AWP is $65.12?

    a. $21.04
    b. $8.02
    c. $13.02
    d. $73.14

CALCULATIONS PRACTICE EXAM

Answers are on page 214.

16. A prescription has been written for Prevacid 30 mg #100, Sig i cap qd, 2 refills; however, the patient's insurance benefit has a 34-day supply limit. If the original prescription is filled for 34 capsules, how many refills of 34 would be available?

    a. 6 refills of 34
    b. 8 refills of 34
    c. 5 refills of 34
    d. 7 refills of 34

17. You are preparing a prescription for Synthroid 0.1 mg tablets. How many micrograms are in each tablet?

    a. 0.1 mg
    b. 0.1 mcg
    c. 100 mg
    d. 100 mcg

18. You are entering a prescription for timolol 0.25% ophthalmic solution 5 ml, Sig i gtt o.u. twice daily. How many days should this bottle last if the dropper delivers 20 drops of timolol 0.25% ophthalmic solution per ml?

    a. 10 days
    b. 50 days
    c. 12.5 days
    d. 25 days

19. The dose of a drug is 250 micrograms per kg of body weight. What dose should be given to a child that weighs 55 lbs?

    a. 6.25 micrograms
    b. 6.25 mg
    c. 12.5 mg
    d. 12.5 micrograms

20. A physician has ordered 15 ml of Brand X Antacid Suspension to be taken four times daily. How many days will a 12 oz. bottle last?

    a. 6 days
    b. 12 days
    c. 3 days
    d. 10 days

Answers are on page 214.

21. How many mcg of digoxin are in 0.4 ml of digoxin solution if the strength of the digoxin solution is 50 mcg per ml?

    a. 20 mcg
    b. 125 mcg
    c. 0.02 mcg
    d. 12.5 mcg

22. You are filling a prescription for gentamicin 80 mg. How much gentamicin solution should be measured from a 2 ml vial of gentamicin 40 mg/ml?

    a. 2 ml
    b. 1 ml
    c. 0.8 ml
    d. 1.6 ml

23. 45 units of Humulin R insulin are to be added to a TPN bag. How much Humulin R (U-100) is needed?

    a. 45 microliters
    b. 0.45 ml
    c. 4.5 ml
    d. 0.45 microliters

24. How much potassium chloride solution (2 mEq/ml) should be added to a 1 liter IV bag if 25 mEq of potassium chloride is needed?

    a. 25 ml
    b. 0.25 ml
    c. 12.5 ml
    d. 50 ml

25. How much sodium chloride is in 25 ml of normal saline?

    a. 225 g
    b. 225 mcg
    c. 225 mg
    d. 2.25 g

CALCULATIONS PRACTICE EXAM

Answers are o page 214.

26. A drug is in a vial that contains 500 mg of the drug in 2 ml of solution. What is the percent strength of this drug?

    a. 2.5%
    b. 25%
    c. 10%
    d. 5%

27. You have dissolved 20 g of drug in 500 ml of solution. What is the percent strength of the resulting solution?

    a. 0.4%
    b. 4%
    c. 0.2%
    d. 2%

28. How many capsules are needed to prepare 30 ml of 1% clindamycin hydrochloride solution if each capsule contains 150 mg of clindamycin hydrochloride?

    a. 4 capsules
    b. 3 capsules
    c. 1 capsule
    d. 2 capsules

29. How much 1% lidocaine is needed to fill an order for 30 mg of lidocaine?

    a. 0.3 ml
    b. 3 ml
    c. 3 microliters
    d. 0.03 ml

30. What is the percent strength of a 1:100 solution?

    a. 10%
    b. 1%
    c. 0.01%
    d. 0.1%

Answers are on page 214.

31. How much gentian violet is needed to prepare 100 ml of a 1:10,000 solution of gentian violet?

    a. 0.01 mg
    b. 10 g
    c. 10 mg
    d. 10 mcg

32. How much vancomycin should be given per dose for a child that weighs 32 lbs if the dose is 10 mg/kg q 6 h IV?

    a. 582 mg
    b. 145 mg
    c. 0.69 mg
    d. 704 mg

33. A patient is to receive 100 mg/kg/day of ampicillin. What is the total daily dose for a patient that weighs 40 lbs?

    a. 182 mg
    b. 1.8 g
    c. 18.2 g
    d. 0.182 g

34. If 250 mg of penicillin VK is equivalent to 400,000 Units of penicillin, how many Units of penicillin are in 1 mg of penicillin VK?

    a. 1,600 U
    b. 1,600 MU
    c. 16 MU
    d. 1.6 U

35. A nomogram has been used to determine a patient's BSA is 1.95. If the dose of a drug is 40 mg/sq. meter, how much drug should be administered per dose?

    a. 780 mg
    b. 7.8 g
    c. 78 mg
    d. 7.8 mg

Answers are on page 214.

36. A 500 ml IV bag is administered over 4 hours. What is the infusion rate?

   a. 125 ml/min
   b. 100 ml/min
   c. 100 ml/hr
   d. 125 ml/hr

37. A 500 ml IV bag is infused at a rate of 100 ml/hr. How long will this bag last?

   a. 2.5 hours
   b. 2 hours
   c. 10 hours
   d. 5 hours

38. An IV has been running at 80 ml/hr for 5 hours and 20 minutes. How much solution has the patient received?

   a. 427 ml
   b. 40 ml
   c. 400 ml
   d. 43 ml

39. An IV is set to deliver 30 drops/min. What is the infusion rate in ml/hr if there are 15 drops/ml?

   a. 30 ml/hr
   b. 40 ml/hr
   c. 120 ml/hr
   d. 270 ml/hr

40. How many ml of a 20% solution should be added to 50 ml of a 40% solution to obtain a 25% solution?

   a. 50 ml
   b. 100 ml
   c. 150 ml
   d. 200 ml

PRACTICE CALCULATION EXAM -- WORKSPACE

Use this space to work out calculations.

ANSWERS TO PRACTICE EXAMS

PRACTICE EXAM

1. b
2. d
3. a
4. a
5. b
6. b
7. b
8. c
9. b
10. c
11. c
12. d
13. d
14. b
15. c
16. a
17. d
18. c
19. d
20. b
21. a
22. d
23. c
24. b
25. c
26. a
27. c
28. c
29. c
30. c
31. a
32. c
33. a
34. d
35. b
36. a
37. a
38. c
39. b
40. c
41. b
42. a
43. c

44. b
45. c
46. b
47. a
48. c
49. b
50. c
51. c
52. b
53. b
54. a
55. b
56. b
57. b
58. b
59. c
60. c
61. d
62. c
63. b
64. b
65. c
66. d
67. a
68. c
69. b
70. c
71. b
72. b
73. c
74. c
75. c
76. b
77. d
78. b
79. b
80. b
81. d
82. c
83. a
84. a
85. b
86. b
87. d

88. a
89. b
90. b
91. a
92. a
93. c
94. d
95. a
96. c
97. d
98. c
99. c
100. b
101. c
102. b
103. c
104. c
105. b
106. c
107. c
108. b
109. c
110. b
111. a
112. d
113. c
114. d
115. b
116. c
117. d
118. b
119. b
120. d
121. a
122. b
123. c
124. d
125. c
126. b
127. a
128. b
129. c
130. d
131. d

132. c
133. c
134. c
135. b
136. d
137. b
138. b
139. b
140. d

CALCULATIONS
PRACTICE EXAM

1. c
2. c
3. b
4. a
5. a
6. d
7. d
8. b
9. c
10. c
11. b
12. b
13. d
14. a
15. a
16. d
17. d
18. d
19. b
20. a
21. a
22. a
23. b
24. c
25. c
26. b
27. b
28. d
29. b
30. b
31. c
32. b

33. b
34. a
35. c
36. d
37. d
38. a
39. c
40. c

ANSWERS TO CHAPTER EXERCISES AND PROBLEMS

CHAPTER 1

p.4
1. Shen Nung
2. salicylic acid
3. materia medica
4. pharmaceutical
5. panacea
6. pharmacology
7. Paracelcus
8. data
9. antitoxin
10. antibiotic
11. hormones
12. human genome
13. OBRA '90
14. formularies
15. managed care

p5.
1. F
2. F
3. T
4. F
5. T
6. T
7. F
8. F
9. T
10. F

p.6
1. c
2. d
3. b
4. a
5. c
6. d
7. b

CHAPTER 2

p.16
1. scope of practice
2. personal inventory
3. confidentiality

4. patient welfare
5. competent
6. certification
7. technicians
8. professionals
9. pharmacist
10. counseling
11. patient rights
12. detail oriented
13. continuing education
14. on-the-job training

p.17
1. T
2. F
3. F
4. T
5. T
6. F
7. F
8. T
9. T
10. F

p.18
1. b
2. d
3. c
4. a
5. b
6. d
7. c
8. b
9. c
10. d

CHAPTER 3

p.24
1. DEA number
2. injunction
3. placebo
4. adverse effect
5. legend drug
6. negligence

ANSWERS TO CHAPTER EXERCISES AND PROBLEMS

CHAPTER 3 CONT'D

7. pediatric
8. labeling
9. "look-alike" regulation
10. liability
11. therapeutic
12. recall
13. controlled substance mark
14. NDC

p.25

1. F
2. F
3. T
4. T
5. T
6. F
7. T
8. T
9. F
10. T

p 26

1. Schedule II
2. Schedule III
3. Class III recall
4. Schedule V
5. Class II recall
6. Schedule I
7. Schedule IV
8. Class I recall

p.27

1. tight, light resistant
2. Endo Labs
3. Endocet
4. Oxycodone and Acetaminophen
5. tablets
6. oxycodone hydrochloride and acetaminophen
7. C-II
8. room temperature
9. 01/00

p.28

1. d
2. a
3. d
4. b
5. c
6. b
7. d
8. c
9. d
10. a

CHAPTER 4

p. 37

1. hypertension
2. thrombosis
3. phlebitis
4. arteriosclerosis
5. cardiomyopathy
6. endocrine
7. hyperlipidemia
8. hypothyroidism
9. somatic
10. anorexia
11. colitis
12. hepatitis
13. gastritis
14. dermatitis
15. subcutaneous
16. transdermal
17. hematoma
18. hemophilia
19. lymphoma
20. leukemia
21. tendinitis
22. neuralgia
23. osteoarthritis
24. endometriosis
25. vaginitis
26. prostatitis
27. bronchitis
28. pulmonary

ANSWERS TO CHAPTER EXERCISES AND PROBLEMS

29. sinusitis
30. cystitis
31. uremia
32. conjunctivitis

p.38
1. a
2. b
3. c
4. d
5. c
6. d
7. b
8. c
9. c
10. b

CHAPTER 5

p.43
1. of each
2. before meals
3. right ear
4. morning
5. left ear
6. before
7. each ear
8. to, up to
9. water
10. add water up to
11. body surface area
12. twice a day
13. with
14. capsules
15. per gastric button
16. dilute
17. dispense
18. per nasogastric tube
19. dextrose 57 in water
20. elixir
21. fluid
22. gram
23. drop
24. hour
25. at bedtime

26. intramuscular
27. intravenous
28. intravenous push
29. no refill
30. intravenous piggyback
31. liter
32. left
33. liquid
34. microgram
35. milliEquivalent
36. milligram
37. milliliter
38. normal saline
39. right eye
40. left eye
41. each eye
42. after meals
43. by mouth
44. as needed
45. each, every
46. every day
47. every 6 hours
48. four times a day
49. a sufficient quantity
50. add sufficient quantity to make
51. without
52. subcutaneously
53. one-half
54. immediately
55. suppository
56. syrup
57. three times a day
58. tablets
59. tablespoon
60. topically
61. teaspoon
62. ointment
63. as directed

p. 46
Prozac Prescription
1. Prozac
2. 20 mg
3. capsules

ANSWERS TO CHAPTER EXERCISES AND PROBLEMS

CHAPTER 5 CONT'D

4. by mouth
5. one capsule every day
6. 2
7. no

Kenalog Prescription
1. 0.1%
2. twice daily

p.47

Protonix Prescription
1. 30
2. 1

Atrovent/Flovent Prescription
1. Each inhaler would last 33 days if two puffs per dose are used or 22 days if three puffs per dose are used. We would normally enter 22 days for the days supply on a prescription of this type.
2. 30 days

p.48

Synthroid Prescription
1. DAW

Miacalcin Prescription
1. Miacalcin is a nasal spray. The directions read "one inhalation every day" and the patient should administer the medication to alternate nostrils, meaning that the patient should not use the same nostril two days in a row.

p.49

Metrogel Prescription
1. A 70 gram tube should be dispensed
2. "per vagina"

Premarin/Provera Prescription
1. Since the patient takes the medication for 21 days and off for 7 days, the medication will last 28 days.
2. Since the patient takes the medication for only 5 days in a 28-day cycle, this medication will also last 28 days.

p.50

Ortho Novum 777 Prescription
1. 7 (1 original fill plus 6 refills)

Bactrim DS Prescription
1. sulfa allergy

p.51

Lorabid Prescription
1. Take one teaspoonful twice daily for 10 days.

Amoxicillin, Biaxin, and Aciphex Prescription
1. 28
2. 14
3. 14

p.52

1. pneumonia, dehydration
2. penicillin allergy
3. every four hours by mouth
4. 2200 and 600 orders
5. 500 mg by mouth, every 12 hours
6. by mouth, each day
7. 8 hours

p.53

1. Lopressor 50 mg, Hydrochlorothiazide 25 mg, and Sonata 5 mg
2. one at bedtime as needed

p.54

Mary Smith Physician Order
1. docusate sodium 100 mg
2. Metamucil

Andrew Smith Physician Order
p.1. This medication should be administered as soon as possible.
2. intramuscular injection

p.55

Steve Smith Physician Order
1. 100 cc per hour
2. hydrochlorothizide 25 mg and Diovan 80 mg

Barbara Smith Physician Order
1. Micronase 5 mg and Ambien 5 mg

ANSWERS TO CHAPTER EXERCISES AND PROBLEMS

2.   Ambien 5 mg

p.56
1.   prescription
2.   extemporaneous compounding
3.   protocols
4.   signa
5.   auxiliary label
6.   medication orders
7.   lookalikes
8.   inscription
9.   DAW
10. Rx
11. institutional labels
12. Schedule II, III, and IV auxiliary label
13. prescription number
14. DEA number

p.57
1.   T
2.   F
3.   F
4.   T
5.   F
6.   T
7.   T
8.   F
9.   F
10. F

p.58
1.   c
2.   b
3.   a
4.   b
5.   b
6.   a
7.   c
8.   c
9.   c
10. c
11. c
12. a
13. b

14. a
15. c

CHAPTER 6

p.62
1.   1.25
2.   0.005
3.   0.75
4.   0.67
5.   0.08
6.   0.425
7.   0.032
8.   0.8%
9.   50%
10. 4.2%
11. 12.5%
12. 7.5%
13. 40%
14. 2.5%

Roman numerals:
15. IV
16. XLIX
17. LXII
18. CVIII
19. XXIV
20. XCVIII
21. XIV
22. 24
23. 104
24. 1200
25. 2 1/2
26. 18
27. 54

p.63, 66-67
1.   40
2.   21
3.   3.5
4.   2400 mg
5.   300 ml
6.   22.5
7.   720

ANSWERS TO CHAPTER EXERCISES AND PROBLEMS

CHAPTER 6 CONT'D

8. 7.2 ml
9. 1.25 ml/min
10. 1.4
11. 360 ml
12. 500 ml 70% dextrose and 500 ml sterile water
13. 285 ml 70% dextrose and 715 ml sterile water
14. 250 ml 50% dextrose and 250 sterile water

p. 68

1.) aminosyn 500 ml
2.) dextrose 400 ml
3.) KCl 12 ml
4.) MVI 5 ml
5.) NaCl 5.45 ml
6.) sterile water 77.55

CHAPTER 7

p.73

1. F
2. T
3. F
4. T
5. F
6. T
7. T
8. T
9. F
10. F

p.74

1. local effect
2. systemic effect
3. degradation
4. adsorb
5. buccal cavity
6. inactive ingredients
7. enteric coated
8. water soluble
9. sublingual administration
10. hemorrhoid

11. parenteral
12. necrosis
13. sterile
14. intradermal injections
15. intravenous sites
16. aqueous
17. solvent
18. trauma
19. colloids
20. emulsions
21. intramuscular injection sites
22. subcutaneous injection sites
23. viscosity
24. biocompatibility
25. wheal
26. lacrimal gland
27. lacrimal canalicula
28. conjunctiva
29. transcorneal transport
30. nasal mucosa
31. atomizer
32. nasal inhaler
33. inspiration
34. metered dose inhalers
35. percutaneous
36. topical
37. hydrates
38. transdermal patches
39. Toxic Shock Syndrome
40. contraceptive
41. IUD

p.76

1. intraocular
2. intranasal
3. sublingual
4. inhalation
5. peroral
6. intravenous
7. vaginal
8. subcutaneous
9. intramuscular

ANSWERS TO CHAPTER EXERCISES AND PROBLEMS

p. 77
1. intradermal
2. subcutaneous
3. intravenous
4. intramuscular

Intramuscular
1. a
2. d
3. b
4. e
5. c

p.78
1. c
2. a
3. b
4. c
5. c
6. b
7. d
8. a
9. a
10. c
11. a
12. d
13. a
14. d

CHAPTER 8

p.83
1. F
2. T
3. T
4. F
5. T
6. F

p.90
1. aseptic techniques
2. pyrogens
3. osmotic pressure
4. isotonic
5. hypertonic

6. hypotonic
7. flow rate
8. heparin lock
9. piggybacks
10. infusion
11. admixture
12. lyophilized
13. diluent
14. ready-to-mix
15. bevel
16. gauge
17. lumen
18. coring
19. membrane filter
20. depth filter
21. final filter
22. laminar flow
23. HEPA filter
24. biological safety hood
25. irrigation solution
26. ampule
27. sharps
28. equivalent weight
29. valence
30. molecular weight
31. ions
32. anhydrous
33. waters of hydration
34. osmosis
35. dialysis

p.92
1. b
2. c
3. a
4. c
5. c
6. c
7. b
8. c
9. a
10. b
11. a
12. a
13. d

ANSWERS TO CHAPTER EXERCISES AND PROBLEMS

CHAPTER 8 CONT'D

14. b
15. c
16. c

CHAPTER 9

p.99
1. F
2. T
3. T
4. F
5. T
6. F
7. F
8. F
9. T
10. T
11. F
12. T

p.104
1. extemporaneous compounding
2. stability
3. anticipatory compounding
4. calibrate
5. volumetric
6. arrest knob
7. meniscus
8. trituration
9. levigation
10. geometric dilution
11. sonication
12. solvent
13. formulation record
14. compounding record
15. syrup
16. sensitivity requirement
17. flocculating agents
18. thickening agent
19. miscible
20. immiscible
21. emulsifier
22. emulsion
23. water-in-oil
24. oil-in-water

25. hydrophilic emulsifier
26. lipophilic emulsifier
27. primary emulsion
28. mucilage
29. compression molding
30. fusion molding
31. "punch" method

p.106
1. a
2. c
3. a
4. c
5. b
6. d
7. b
8. b
9. a
10. a
11. a
12. d
13. d
14. b
15. b
16. c

CHAPTER 10

p.113
1. T
2. T
3. T
4. F
5. F
6. T
7. T
8. F
9. F
10. T
11. F

p.114
1. biopharmaceutics
2. site of action
3. receptor
4. selective action

Answers to Chapter Exercises and Problems

5.   agonists
6.   antagonists
7.   minimum effective concentration
8.   onset of action
9.   therapeutic window
10. disposition
11. passive diffusion
12. active transport
13. hydrophobic
14. hydrophilic
15. lipoidal
16. gastric emptying time
17. complex
18. protein binding
19. metabolite
20. enzyme
21. enzyme induction
22. enzyme inhibition
23. first pass metabolism
24. enterohepatic cycling
25. nephron
26. glomerular filtration
27. bioavailability
28. bioequivalency
29. pharmaceutical equivalents
30. pharmaceutical alternative
31. therapeutic equivalents

p.116
1.   b
2.   c
3.   c
4.   b
5.   a
6.   a
7.   c
8.   d
9.   b
10. d
11. a
12. c
13. a
14. b

CHAPTER 11

p.120
1.   hypersensitivity
2.   anaphylactic shock
3.   idiosyncrasy
4.   hepatotoxicity
5.   nephrotoxicity
6.   carcinogenicity
7.   teratogenicity
8.   additive effects
9.   synergism
10. inhibition
11. displacement
12. antidote
13. drug-diet interactions
14. hypothyroidism
15. hyperthyroidism
16. hepatic disease
17. cirrhosis
18. acute viral hepatitis

p.121
1.   F
2.   T
3.   T
4.   T
5.   T
6.   F
7.   T
8.   F
9.   T
10. T

p.122
1.   d
2.   b
3.   c
4.   c
5.   c
6.   d
7.   a
8.   d
9.   a

ANSWERS TO CHAPTER EXERCISES AND PROBLEMS

CHAPTER 11 CONT'D

10. b
11. a
12. b
13. b

CHAPTER 12

p.126
1. primary literature
2. tertiary literature
3. abstracting services
4. Material Safety Data Sheets
5. secondary literature
6. American Hospital Formulary Service
7. Drug Facts and Comparisons
8. USP DI
9. Handbook on Injectable Drugs
10. World Wide Web
11. modem
12. browser
13. Internet service provider
14. URL

p.127
1. F
2. T
3. T
4. F
5. F
6. T
7. F
8. T
9. F
10. T
11. T

p.128
1. c
2. b
3. b
4. d
5. c
6. a
7. c

8. a
9. a
10. c
11. a
12. c
13. c
14. d

CHAPTER 13

p.132
1. open formulary
2. closed formulary
3. turnover
4. Schedule II substances
5. perpetual inventory
6. point of sale system
7. reorder points
8. order entry device
9. database
10. purchase order number
11. stock bottles
12. unit-dose
13. dispensing units

p.133
1. T
2. F
3. T
4. F
5. T
6. F
7. T
8. F
9. F
10. T

p.134
1. b
2. d
3. b
4. c
5. a
6. a
7. c

8. c
9. d
10. b

CHAPTER 14

p.138
1. pharmacy benefits managers
2. online adjudication
3. co-insurance
4. co-pay
5. dual co-pay
6. maximum allowable cost
7. U&C or UCR
8. HMO
9. POS
10. PPO
11. deductible
12. prescription drug benefit cards
13. patient identification number
14. Medicare
15. Medicaid
16. CMS 1500 form (formerly HCFA 1500)
17. workers' compensation
18. patient assistance programs
19. universal claim form

p.139
1. F
2. T
3. T
4. T
5. F
6. T
7. F
8. T

p.140
1. b
2. a
3. d
4. b
5. d
6. b
7. d
8. c

9. b
10. d

CHAPTER 15

p.146
1. OBRA '90
2. interpersonal skills
3. scope of practice
4. confidentiality
5. refrigeration
6. patient identification number
7. group number
8. signa
9. DEA number
10. safety caps
11. counting tray
12. shelf stickers
13. bar code
14. auxiliary labels
15. unit price

p.147
1. T
2. T
3. T
4. F
5. F
6. T
7. F
8. T
9. T
10. F
11. T

p.148
1. b
2. a
3. c
4. b
5. a
6. a
7. c
8. c
9. b
10. c

ANSWERS TO CHAPTER EXERCISES AND PROBLEMS

CHAPTER 16

p.154
1. Nurse Practitioner
2. Registered Nurse, R.N.
3. Licensed Practical Nurse, L.P.N.
4. unit dose
5. standing order
6. PRN order
7. STAT order
8. medication administration record (MAR)
9. code carts
10. centralized pharmacy system
11. inpatient pharmacy
12. decentralized pharmacy system
13. formulary
14. clean rooms
15. outpatient pharmacy
16. policy and procedure manual
17. distributive pharmacist
18. consultant pharmacist
19. automated dispensing system

p.155
1. F
2. F
3. T
4. T
5. F
6. T
7. T

p.156
1. b
2. b
3. d
4. a
5. a
6. d
7. d
8. b
9. c
10. b
11. b
12. c

CHAPTER 17

p.159
1. F
2. T
3. F
4. T
5. F
6. F
7. T
8. T

p.160
1. d
2. d
3. d
4. a
5. a
6. c
7. d
8. c
9. a
10. b

APPENDIX A

p.176
1. Analgesic
2. Respiratory Agent
3. Cardiovascular Agent
4. Anti-infective
5. Anti-infective
6. Analgesic
7. Cardiovascular Agent
8. Anti-infective
9. Musculoskeletal Agent
10. Anti-infective
11. Gastrointestinal Agent
12. Anti-infective
13. Anti-infective
14. Dermatological Agent
15. Antineoplastic
16. Cardiovascular Agent
17. Gastrointestinal Agent
18. Cardiovascular Agent
19. Anti-infective

20. Cardiovascular Agent
21. Antidiabetic
22. Cardiovascular Agent
23. Dermatological Agent
24. Analgesic
25. Antidiabetic
26. Respiratory Agent
27. Gastrointestinal Agent
28. Gastrointestinal Agent
29. Gastrointestinal Agent
30. Cardiovascular Agent
31. Cardiovascular Agent
32. Cardiovascular Agent
33. Cardiovascular Agent
34. Cardiovascular Agent
35. Anesthetic
36. Gastrointestinal Agent
37. Gastrointestinal Agent
38. Electrolytic Agent
39. Analgesic
40. Dermatological Agent
41. Electrolytic Agent
42. Antineoplastic
43. Anesthetic
44. Analgesic
45. Gastrointestinal Agent
46. Anti-infective
47. Cardiovascular Agent
48. Cardiovascular Agent

KEY CONCEPTS INDEX

The following lists the topics found in the Key Concepts sections of this workbook.

KEY CONCEPTS INDEX